MASSAGE

MASSAGE
The Oriental Method

Katsusuke Serizawa, M.D.
Professor at the Tokyo University of Education

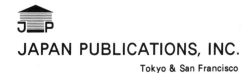

JAPAN PUBLICATIONS, INC.

Tokyo & San Francisco

THIS IS A POPULAR VERSION OF *MASSAGE: THE ORIENTAL METHOD*
BY THE SAME AUTHOR AND PUBLISHERS.

Library of Congress Catalog Card Number 73-188762
ISBN 0-87040-168-8

JAPAN PUBLICATIONS, INC.
JAPAN PUBLICATIONS TRADING COMPANY
1255 Howard Street, San Francisco, Calif. 94103 U.S.A.
P.O. Box 5030 Tokyo International, Tokyo, Japan
First Printing: July, 1972
Second Printing: October, 1972
Third Printing: May, 1973

Layout and Typography by Soshichi Toyoshima
Photographys by Tokiharu Ichimura
Printed in Japan

Preface

The smoke, smog, noise, and congestion of modern urban life exerts far-reaching influences on the human body. For example overheated rooms in winter and chilly air-conditioned ones in summer bring on headaches, dizziness, ringing in the ears, stiff shoulders, pains in the back, constipation, stomach disorders, chill in the hands and feet, numbness, insomnia, sluggishness, and a number of other minor but troublesome ailments. On examining a patient suffering from one or more of these distresses, a doctor trained in the Western medical tradition generally reports that nothing serious seems to be the trouble, still the patient goes on feeling the symptoms.

Because Western medicine has tended to overlook minor complaints of this kind, many people all over the world are now turning for help to oriental treatment methods, especially Chinese medicine, *amma* massage, acupuncture, moxa, and *shiatsu* massage.

All of these treatments originated in China and, traveling through the Korean Peninsula to Japan, have undergone centuries of refinement to reach the stage where today they can offer surprisingly effective relief from the complaints mentioned in the preceding paragraph. All of these kinds of treatment are based on the functioning of the internal organs and the nervous system. This book, too, explains oriental massage as a way of performing certain operations on the vital points called *tsubo* to bring about relief from a number of ailments.

The policy of the text and layout is to make it possible for members of the family to massage each other in a friendly and relaxing way. For this reason text, charts, and photographs have been used together to enable the reader to understand the treatment methods quickly and completely. In addition to general oriental massage, I have included a brief section on the more specialized shiatsu system and its effects.

Oriental massage depends for its effectiveness on the theory of nerve nodules, which are called tsubo. So that the reader may understand why this system of massage works, I have explained tsubo and their actions in the first three chapters. Because this theory is basic to all oriental medicine and treatment, I urge the reader to read the explanations thoroughly. With a firm knowledge of the tsubo, one may go on quickly to study the basic massage techniques and their applications.

In a recent trip through twenty-two major cities in twelve nations I examined clinical rehabilitation methods and learned that in both East and West, natural treatment without equipment or medicine—in short, traditional Japanese treatment—has become a subject of great interest and considerable admiration. I have resolved to write a book on this important subject not because I want to demonstrate my own skills at massage treatment. On the contrary, my sole interest is in presenting to the Westerner one way of breaking free of therapy dependent totally on machines and of returning to an essentially human kind of treatment. I am convinced that this is the kind of medicine that can help save mankind from the isolation and inhumanity of the modern condition.

In connection with the publication of this book I should like to express my sincerest thanks to the Japan Publications, Inc., and their editorial department, to Soshichi Toyoshima and Yukishige Takahashi of the same company who devoted much time and thought to the preparation of text and layout, to the translator Richard L. Gage, and to the photographer, Tokiharu Ichimura.

Spring, 1972

KATSUSUKE SERIZAWA

Contents

Chapter 1
The Philosophy of Oriental Medicine

The Origin

First of all for the sake of clarity, I must say that the term "oriental medicine" is in fact too broad to be strictly meaningful, but I use it in a special—and today generally accepted—sense to mean medicine that originated in China and traveled to Japan by way of Korea. Chinese medicine—or *Kampo*—may be divided into two major streams of development. Therapeutical systems arising in the area of the Yellow River include acupuncture, moxa, and amma massage, all of which are widely practiced today in Japan.

Primitive origins of acupuncture and moxa are closely related to the nature of the land in the Yellow River district. The soil there is infertile. Though rocks and boulders abound, vegetation is generally of the small grass kind and includes the plant known as mugwort. Consequently, in the distant past when people there injured themselves in such a way that pus formed, it was only natural that they use small splinters of stone to prick the wound to discharge the suppuration. Similarly, when some other bodily part failed to perform as it ought to, they applied small amounts of dried mugwort to the affected area and lit it. The localized heat generated by the burning material gave relief from their ailments. In these ways, acupuncture and moxa developed.

The amma massage method grew from the simple habit of pressing or rubbing numbed or chilled hands and feet with the fingers and palms of the hands. Over many long ages of practical experience with these treatments, the Chinese people learned the spots on the body where acupuncture, moxa, and massage produce maximum effect. These are the tsubo or vital points that will be the subject of my further discussion.

In contrast to this northern branch of Chinese medicine, the southern region around the Yangtze River produced its own system. It too is based on the nature of the land. In the southern zone of China the land is rich, and plants of all kinds grow in profusion. When the primitive inhabitants of this area fell ill, they concocted medicinal preparations from the dried roots of

1

plants and the barks of trees. For some time the two systems existed side by side without any significant interpenetration, but when the Han dynasty (206 B.C. to A.D. 220) unified the nation, the two were blended to produce what is today called *Kampo* or Chinese medicine. (The *Kam* part of the word is a phonetic variation of *kan*, the Japanese reading of the character used to write the name of the Han dynasty.)

Chinese medicine of this compound kind first entered Japan in the sixth century (Asuka period) and was the main medical stream from that time until the end of the Edo period (1615-1868). After the beginning of the Meiji period (1868-1912), Western influences flooded the nation. With them came Western medicine, which replaced Chinese medicine as the primary field of treatment and research. Nonetheless, Chinese medicine continues to be popular with the people. It is in fact widely practiced today.

Internal Organs

Chinese medical thought categorizes internal organs into two groups. The first set, consisting of five organs—most accurately six, but I shall have more to say on this subject later—is called *Zo*. Six others organs are called *Fu*. But to explain these categories, it is important to sketch in the cosmological system on which the system is founded.

Oriental medicine, a fundamentally simple system, follows the path of nature as interpreted in oriental philosophy. First, all natural phenomena belong to one of two big groups: the yin, or negative phenomena, and the yang, or positive ones. These phenomena may be further divided into groups according to their physical composition; that is all of them are plant, heat, earth, mineral, or liquid. This five oriental elements are symbolized as wood, fire, earth, metal, and water.

Human beings, too, as part of the natural world, conform to these general rules. The male is yang or positive and the female is yin or negative. The Zo and Fu organs that make up the human body fit into the same system. Finally, just as a tree buds in the spring, puts forth leaves in the summer, bears fruit in the fall, and withers in the winter, so human beings are born, experience a period of maximum activity, bear young, grow old, and die.

All of the symptoms of illness too belong to this natural cycle. Therefore, unlike Western medicine, which immediately attaches names to symptoms and categorizes them according to kinds of illnesses, the medicine of the Orient regards them as strictly natural phenomena and treats them for themselves alone.

The yang-yin, male-female human body becomes in effect a small world of nature governed —as is the larger world of nature— by the five elements wood, fire, earth, metal, and water. These elements are represented by the five Zo internal organs: the liver represents wood; the heart, fire; the spleen, earth, the lungs, metal; and the kidneys, water. Here it is important to give a word of caution to the reader. These translations of oriental terms are not entirely accurate for this reason. In the light of modern Western medical thought, words like "heart," "lungs," etc., stand for very definite physical things. Though the words used in oriental medicine are the same, they do not always signify the same things. In reading this explanation, attempt to divorce yourself from Western medical thought.

As important as they are, the Zo organs alone cannot manage all the complicated functions of the body. They require assistance from a group of organs called the Fu. The Zo and the Fu organs work in complementary pairs. The assistant organ of the liver, for example, is the gall bladder. Incidentally, even modern medical science recognizes a close relationship between these two organs. The gall bladder lies below and collects the bile produced by the liver. The small intestine is the complementary Fu organ of the heart, and the stomach works together with what I am calling the spleen. In fact, the oriental term for the spleen is closer in meaning to the pancreas. Once again modern science shows that the pancreas, located directly behind the heart, bears an inseparable relation to that organ. Finally, the large intestine complements the lungs, and the urinary bladder the kidneys.

These then are the five major combinations of organs that control the functioning of the human body. As I said earlier, however, traditionally there are six such pairs. The sixth Zo organ is a protective sack that the ancients believed must be present to protect the heart, the most vital of all organs. The sixth Fu, the complement of the protective sack, is called the triple-heat. As long as there is life in the body, it is warm. For this reason Chinese of long ago presupposed some source of this heat. This they called the triple-heat, or *sansho* in Japanese.

I am aware that from the Western scientific standpoint the six combinations seem strange. But in dealing with oriental medicine, one must remember that the terms represent the operations that control the life activities of the body in relation to the world of nature. In other words, though autopsy might not reveal the existence of these organs as described here, they nonetheless do exist as oriental medical principles. Western science is based on the rational examination of analyzable facts. Whatever does not fit the rational approach is ruthlessly discarded. But is it not true that over-emphasis on rationalism has led the world to the present state of environmental pollution and drug abuse? The oriental tradition, on the other hand, adopts the view that even the bodily organs that we take for granted constitute something miraculous and unfathomable, something, in other words, that does not lend itself to the clarity demanded of purely rational thinking.

Oriental medicine attempts to deal with this "something miraculous" on its own terms. In consequence, it makes no attempt to force the mutual relations among all body parts into rational patterns by excessive divisions of organs into analyzable entities. The theory of the six Zo and six Fu organs is the pervading theme of all its therapy.

Chapter 2
Tsubo on the Human Body

Keiraku Energy Systems

Since the human body is completely controlled by the Zo and Fu internal organs, when one of these is in some way impaired the microcosm of human activity loses its harmony and drive. Oriental medicine posits a circulation system of the energy produced to regulate these vitally important organs. Called *keiraku*—for reasons I shall explain soon—these systems are the basis of oriental therapy. According to this line of thought, the body from the top of the head to the tips of the feet, is divided into a horizontal and a vertical system of energy: the former is called the *kei* and the latter the *raku*. Each of them is subdivided into minor systems named for the organ that the energy system controls: 1. lung kei, 2. large intestine kei, 3. stomach kei, 4. spleen kei, 5. heart kei, 6. small intestine kei, 7. bladder kei, 8. kidney kei, 9. protective sack kei, 10. triple-heat kei, 11. gall bladder kei, 12. liver kei (see pp. 6-11).

In addition there is a raku system for each of these twelve organs. The systems begin at the lungs—lung kei and lung raku—and follow in the order given, ending at the liver kei and raku. The systems then return to the lungs; in other words, all of the kei and raku systems in the body are interconnected to form one large energy-supply system that, as long as it functions properly, keeps the body in good health.

In addition to these twelve, however, there are eight control keiraku systems that cross the body horizontally, vertically, and diagonally. These are called the *kikei* ranges. The most important of them, the two systems that constantly control the flows of energy through the twelve keiraku systems, are the *ninmyaku* system, which begins at the center of the face, passes to the chest, and then through the abdomen; and the *tokumyaku* system, which begins in the buttocks, crosses up the back and spinal column, then the rear of the neck and the head.

Finally, the Chinese philosophy of medicine assigns positive (yang) significance and names to the keiraku systems and symptoms associated with the six Zo organs and negative (yin) significance to those of the six Fu organs.

5

LUNG KEI

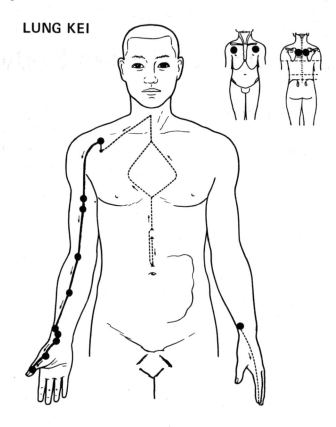

LARGE INTESTINE KEI

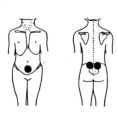

——————— Keiraku on the body surface
················· Keiraku within the body
●   Major tsubo

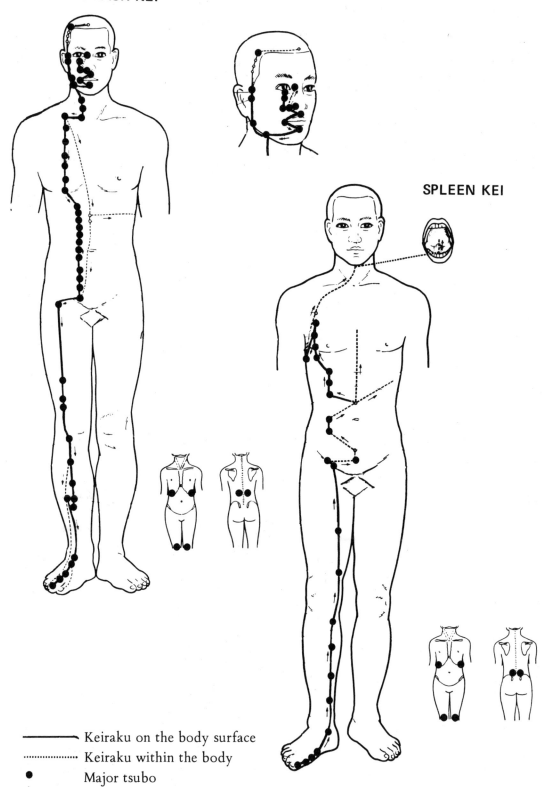

STOMACH KEI

SPLEEN KEI

——————— Keiraku on the body surface

··············· Keiraku within the body

● Major tsubo

HEART KEI

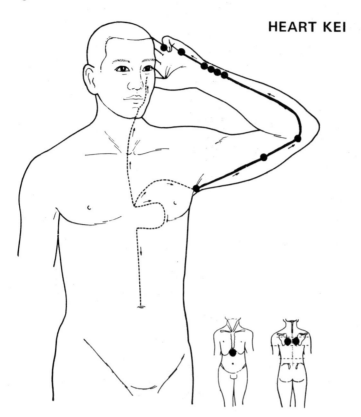

SMALL INTESTINE KEI

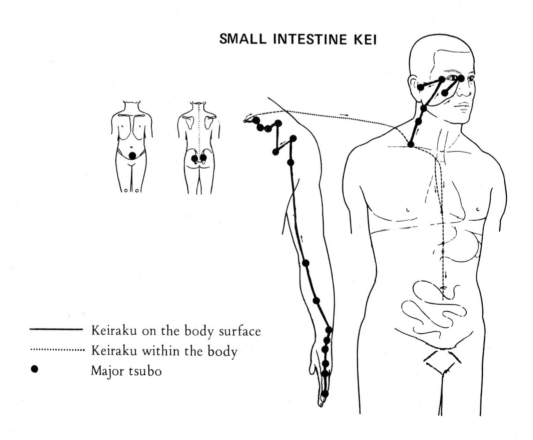

————— Keiraku on the body surface
················ Keiraku within the body
● Major tsubo

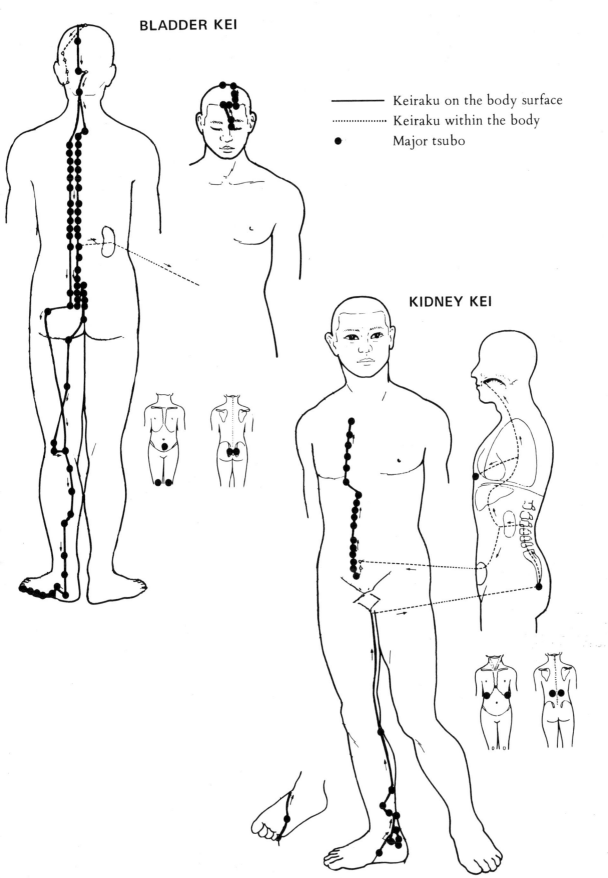

BLADDER KEI

Keiraku on the body surface
Keiraku within the body
Major tsubo

KIDNEY KEI

PROTECTIVE SACK KEI

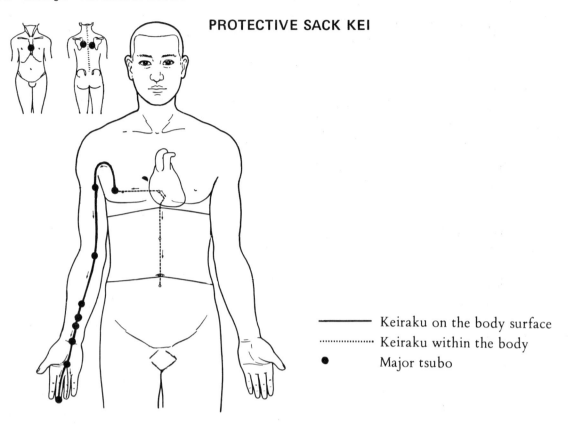

——————— Keiraku on the body surface
·············· Keiraku within the body
● Major tsubo

TRIPLE HEART KEI

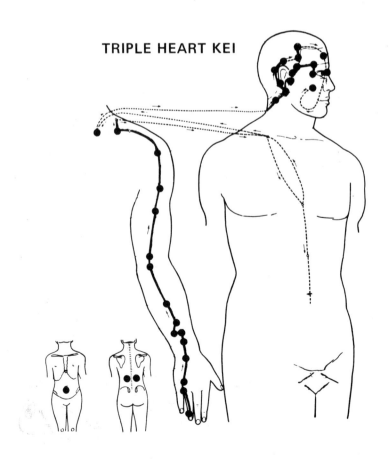

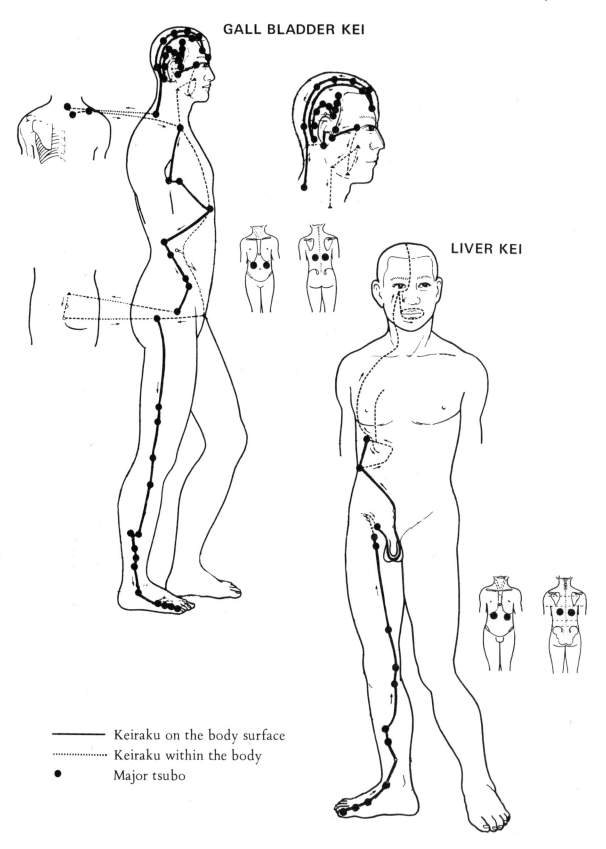

GALL BLADDER KEI

LIVER KEI

——————— Keiraku on the body surface
·················· Keiraku within the body
● Major tsubo

Locations of the Tsubo

I have gone into some detail about the basic keiraku energy systems of the body because these are the systems along which lie the 365 tsubo, or vital points, of the human body. Now I must explain the locations of these tsubo and go into the way in which it is possible to diagnose disorders and to treat them by applying pressure on these tsubo.

The chart on this page shows the twelve front and twelve rear tsubo on the human body. If pressure applied to these points produces pain, there is a disorder in the Zo and Fu organs associated with that tsubo and with the associated keiraku system.

A group of physicians once performed a clinical experiment on fifty healthy persons and fifty patients suffering from various disorders to see if there is a connection between Western rational medicine and ancient Chinese practices. The results of electrical-resistance skin tests, electromyograms, and pulse-wave tests showed that—with allowances for certain individual differences—patients with the various disorders exhibited concentrations of muscular change in the tsubo associated with the organs in which the disorders occurred.

To determine the keiraku system requiring massage treatment, press on the points shown in the right chart. If pain occurs when pressure is applied to point 1 on the front of the body, the trouble is in the lung keiraku system. If pain occurs at point 2 on the front of the body, the trouble is in the large intestine keiraku, and so forth. In the explanations, each tsubo is said to be located at a certain place. Of course, they are not in exact locations in all people. Allowance must be made for the individual human being and for the illness in question.

For that reason, to find the place requiring treatment, it is essential to press lightly in the generally vicinity of the tsubo as described in the text. You will soon come to a tight and very sensitive spot. This is the tsubo by treating which you will bring relief of pain and discomfort. To make the locations of the tsubo easier to understand, I have included charts of the human skeletal and musculatory systems on pp. 14-15.

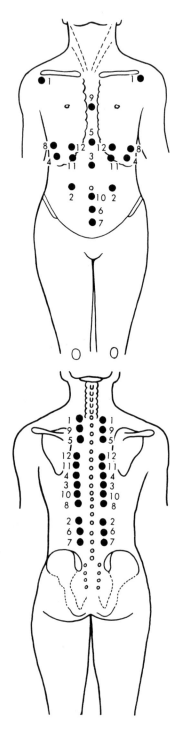

Relation between Tsubo and Bodily Disorders

Why do bodily disorders produce changes in the tsubo, and why does treatment at those points bring relief? According to oriental medical theory, disorders arise when the energy flow in the keiraku systems I have already explained breaks down in one way or another. For instance, when one of the Zo or Fu organs functions sluggishly, the energy flow throughout the body slows down. This phenomenon resembles the breaking of a flow of water caused by stepping on the hose through which the water is traveling. The tsubo are located along the keiraku energy-control systems at places where the flow can easily become stagnant. Therefore, by pressing, rubbing, or massaging the tsubo, the energy flow is improved, and the symptoms are relieved.

The tsubo themselves are the places on the body where stagnation of energy produces a number of phenomena. At this point, I must again remind the reader that this energy system, as well as the keiraku themselves and the Zo and Fu organs, are not recognized by modern Western medical science as having a physical existence in the human body. We in the Orient, however, make use of these principles in therapy. As I have said, oriental medicine gives first consideration to the symptoms. Western medical science, on the other hand, has progressed through dissection and physiology to develop a pathological theory based on the structures and functions of the human body. From this it has produced diagnostic therapy. Oriental medicine followed a different path: it first treats the symptoms and, from a knowledge of them, develops the theory of the Zo and Fu organs and the keiraku systems.

As a case in point, if one examines a part of the body where there are sensations of pain, chill, flushing, stiffness, or collapse one will notice that the skin in that zone is very rough and dry. Suitable secretions of oil and sweat generally keep the skin smooth and pliant, but it becomes rough and dry when the secretions of these two substances fall below a certain level. This condition is proof that discord has arisen in the autonomic nervous system, which controls circulation, respiration, digestion, reproduction, and secretion.

THE HUMAN SKELETON

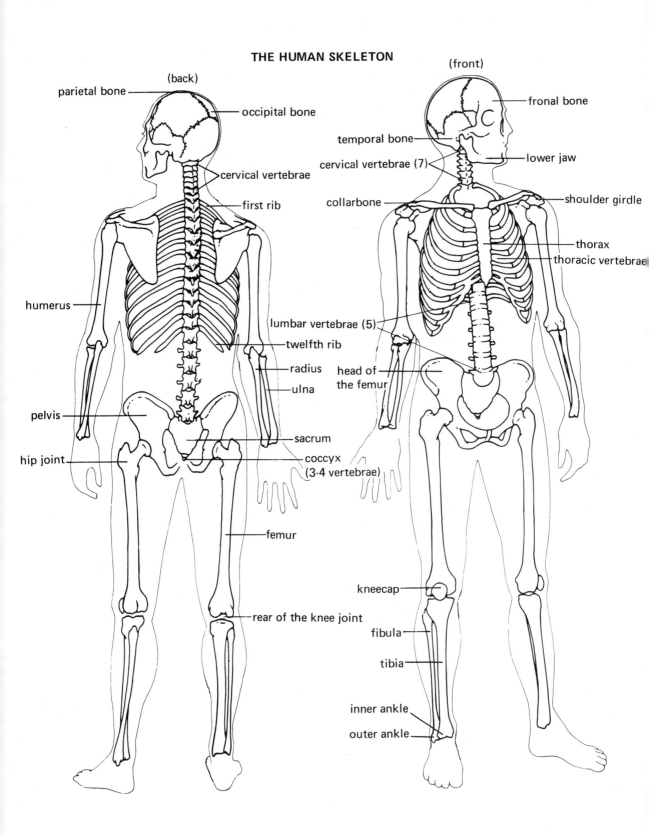

(back)

(front)

parietal bone

occipital bone

cervical vertebrae

first rib

humerus

lumbar vertebrae (5)

twelfth rib

radius

ulna

pelvis

sacrum

hip joint

coccyx
(3-4 vertebrae)

femur

rear of the knee joint

fronal bone

temporal bone

cervical vertebrae (7)

lower jaw

collarbone

shoulder girdle

thorax

thoracic vertebrae

head of
the femur

kneecap

fibula

tibia

inner ankle

outer ankle

HUMAN MUSCULATURE

(front)

(back)

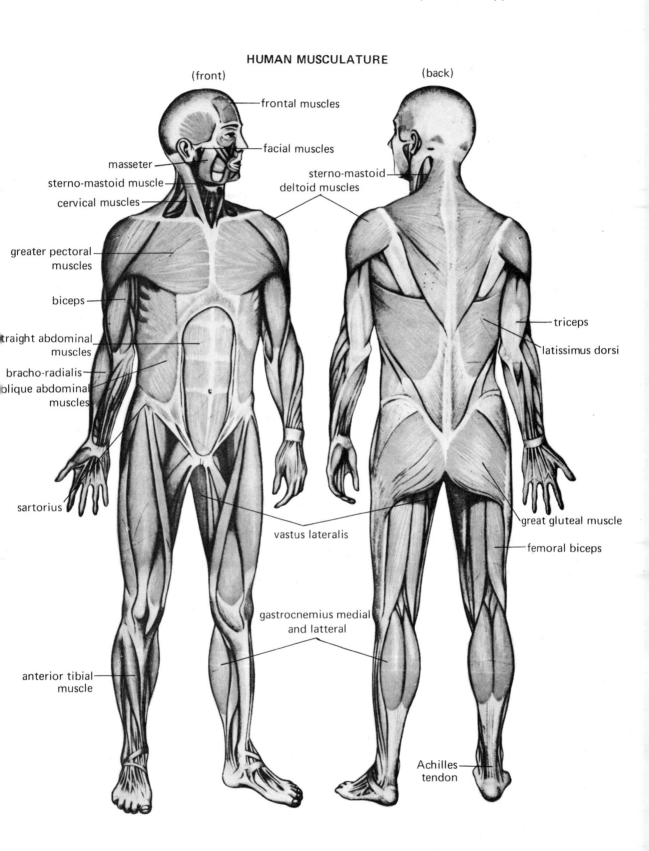

frontal muscles

facial muscles

masseter

sterno-mastoid muscle

cervical muscles

sterno-mastoid

deltoid muscles

greater pectoral muscles

biceps

straight abdominal muscles

bracho-radialis

oblique abdominal muscles

sartorius

vastus lateralis

triceps

latissimus dorsi

great gluteal muscle

femoral biceps

gastrocnemius medial and latteral

anterior tibial muscle

Achilles tendon

Consequently, by finding the tsubo in the area where the skin is dry and rough, it is possible to determine which of the Zo or Fu organs associated with the system in that part of the body is out of order.

To return to oriental treatment, however, I must point out that since the tsubo is the point on the keiraku system where energy tends to stagnate, its location and that of the afflicted organ need not be close to each other. For example, some patients are startled to learn that the proper tsubo for treatment of haemorrhoids is located on the top of the head. Nevertheless, this is the case. The reason massage and shiatsu are effective in relieving pain is that they use an entirely different stimulus from an entirely different direction to counter a distress signal transmitted along the nerves from the brain. Electrophysiology experiments have proven that in this way it is possible to normalize such signals from the brain.

Furthermore, electromyograms, photoelectric transistors for the recording of pulse waves, and tests on the electro-resistance of the skin have shown that such symptoms as chilling, flushing, and stiffness resulting from blood flow and muscular conditions can be relieved by the application of stimulus. Daily experiments in my laboratory have shown that stimulus on the pertinent tsubo can relieve symptoms caused by abnormalities in the body organization and internal organs. Furthermore, this has the effect of returning the entire body functioning apparatus to normal.

Currently, study is being made to determine whether the belief that injections are more effective when given at one of the tsubo is founded in fact. A number of other university clinical laboratories in many parts of the world are conducting similar research. In conclusion, I hope that in these pages I have shown that far from being mystic and miraculous, oriental medicine is a scientific therapy based on experience.

Chapter 3
Why Tsubo Therapy Works

Current Experiments on the Nature of the Tsubo

Only in this century did experimental research and clinical study of oriental medical therapy get under way. Earlier, it had been considered mystic or strange. Because of the relatively recent development of such study, theories about the true nature of oriental medicine are not yet adequately organized and systematized.

For instance, some schools of modern medical thought regard the keiraku and the tsubo as a system of nerve reflexes connecting internal organs and the body wall. The energy circulation system of the Zo and Fu organs is thought of as a unified function separate from that of the blood circulatory and the nervous system. Dr. Bonhan Kim of the Pyongyang University in Korea claims to have identified an actual physical system connecting the tsubo within the organization of the human body. He is currently carrying out further study of what he calls the Bonhan vessels and the Bonhan small bodies.

At this point I shall explain the tsubo therapy method in terms of modern medical theories of nerve reflexes and from the oriental medical clinical standpoint; but before doing so, I must say that I base my interpretation and applications of the many theories concerning this system on my own long years of clinical experience and research. I do not, on the other hand, imply that any one interpretation or application is the only outstanding one. All that I assert is the clinical validity of the system I shall describe as I have used it in my own practice.

Surface Manifestation of Organic Disorders

Among the nervous reflex systems of the human body, one of the most representative is the mechanism whereby organic disorders are made manifest on skin, muscle, and subdermal organizations that have nerve connections with the afflicted inner part. These surface parts of the body constantly receive stimuli from the brain and spinal column by way of the network of nerves that extends over the entire body. When one of the inner organs is out of order, the centripetal impulses flowing from it and those flowing from the skin, muscles, and subdermal regions encounter each other, join, and set up a reflex phenomenon. The symptom occurs at the level on the spinal column where nerves associated with the afflicted organ are located. These reflex phenomena may be divided into three large categories: sensory, motor, and autonomic.

In the case of the first, an organic disorder sends to the spinal chord centripetal impulses unlike the ordinary ones. When this happens the nerves at the levels of the individual vertebrae become oversensitized. Slight external stimuli on the skin near the affected vertebrae produce pain or numbness, when similar pressure under ordinary situations would result in no discomfort. The influence is especially strong on skin, subdermal organizations (united bodies), and muscles located not far below the skin where the sensory nerves are highly developed.

Disorders in organs connected with motor nerves produce tension or contraction in spots, clusters, or bands in muscles located near the body surface. Among these manifestations, all of which affect a limited area, are so-called stiff shoulders, back, arms, and legs. In these cases, the body attempts to protect the ailing interior part by stiffening and hardening outer parts. But when the impulses from the disordered interior organ become very strong, the stiffening of the muscles can spread beyond localized spots, clusters, and bands and advance to a stage where physical therapy of the kind described in this book is ineffectual. The stiffening of the entire abdomen in cases of acute appendicitis is a case in point.

The final of the three categories involves manifestations of organic disorder in the bodily functions controlled by the autonomic nervous system, especially in those related to the secretion of sweat and oil in the skin and the blood vessels supplying these areas. Such manifestations take the form of dry, scaly skin caused by irregularities in the secretion of sweat and oil and of gooseflesh. When the blood vessels fail to function normally, the skin becomes either cold or flushed and overheated. Doctor Yoshio Nakatani, of the Osaka Medical University, has spent a great deal of time studying the effects of impulses from internal organs on dermal oil secretion and has discovered that some of the surface muscle bands and tsubo are excellent electricity conductors and are very effective in treating a variety of symptoms.

Futhermore, our laboratory in cooperation with the physical therapy laboratory of Tokyo University, has studied variations in electrical flow over the surface of the body. As long as the human body is alive, it is influenced by electrical currents from outside. Though the quantities of this electrical current are minute, our study has shown that its flow sometimes stops and that places where it tends to stagnate are connected with a variety of internal disorders and abnormalities.

Stimulating the Surface of the Body to Correct Internal Organs

Since, as I have shown, internal abnormalities exert an influence on the surface of the body, it is naturally possible to influence internal organs by means of stimuli on the body surface. For example, by applying stimulus to a part of the surface of the body, it is possible to stimulate the spinal chord and other nerves controlled by the same level of the central nervous core. It has been scientifically proven that such stimulus sets up sensory and motor activities in internal organs, influences blood vessels and capillaries, and produces changes in secretions of hormones. In fact, in our laboratory, we have used x-rays to show that heat stimulus on the tsubo of the back reduces the size of the gall bladder, whereas heat treatment on the tsubo of the toes increases it. In short, when an irregularity occurs in the functioning of the internal organizations or organs, stimulus to the part of the body surface related to the pertinent internal organ corrects the trouble.

Finding the Correct Tsubo

Having explained in general how stimuli to the body surface relieve symptoms of internal disorder, I must discuss locating the tsubo, or spots on the body where pressure, acupuncture, moxa, or other health therapies must be applied. By and large, the explanations in the individual chapters and the charts on pages

10-14 reveal the locations of the tsubo, but I shall here give a short simple explanation of the basic way to locate them.

Using the charts on pages 10-14, roughly locate a certain tsubo and then find its position more accurately by applying three diagnostic methods: touch, squeeze, and press. Of course none of these actions is performed with violence. Touches are made several times in the general area of the tsubo. Squeezing is done lightly three or four times with the thumbs and index fingers. Finally pressing is light; it may be done with the thumbs or with the fingers.

In touching the person's body, use both hands—either fingers or palms—and touch both sides of the body with equal pressure. If there is nothing wrong with the patient's condition, the feel of his body on both sides will seem the same. Moreover pressure applied to both sides will affect him in the same way. But if the feel of the skin is not the same on both sides, an internal disorder is manifesting itself on the body surface.

For instance, the examiner might feel as if one of his hands is not coming into direct contact with the skin—almost as if that hand were gloved and the other naked. This suggests that the sensory nerves in the area are dulled. If, however, the skin on one side of the body is much more sensitive than that on the other, the sensory nerves are over-sensitized. Next, to find the subdermal area affected by the internal disorder, lightly squeeze both sides of the body in the same way and with the same degree of pressure. The affected zone will feel different to the examiner, and in the majority of cases it will be either very sensitive or numb. Finally, by pressing the area that is now established as abnormal, it is possible to locate the part of the body where the pain actually occurs. It may be the unified bodies under the skin, the membranes encasing the muscles beneath these bodies, or—still deeper—the muscles, which may be stiff or contracted. The stiffened muscular areas may occur as spots, clusters, or bands depending on the case in question.

By applying this three-stage diagnostic method, one may find out first the sensitive part of the skin, then the affected sub-dermal organizations, and lastly the muscle that is in pain. In the initial stage of examination, there are certain important clues to the location of the tsubo. The skin in the vicinity of the affected part may be cold or flushed, it may be dry or wrinkled, or it may show an abundance of freckles or a rash.

Chapter 4

Practical Massage Techniques

Among the practical massage techniques explained in this book, tsubo therapy is the most important. In compiling this work I have concentrated on the methods that can be performed at home by anyone in the hope that I will thus be able to contribute to the prompt and effective relief of those painful symptoms that often make life miserable.

Amma, or pressure and rubbing massage, is one of the traditional therapeutical methods of oriental medicine. In the past—and this is true to some extent today—amma has been considered an occupation for the blind. This massage method calms irritated nerves and normalizes sluggish bodily functions. In short, by pressing and rubbing the muscular areas around the tsubo and sometimes moving the bodily joints, one may use amma to keep the body healthy and strong.

In the past, amma techniques fell into three major categories. Rubbing and pressure were used to restore the body to normal functioning. In the second category the fingers and palms of the hands were employed to limber and refresh tired and stiff muscles all over the body. The third method involved thorough exercise of the joints. With the Meiji Restoration of 1868, however, Western-style massage along with a flood of other Western influences entered Japan. When this happened, amma was related to the function of relieving tired muscles only, and Western massage became the major therapeutic system of its kind.

The Japanese, however, were soon to discover that traditional amma and massage based on Western medical theories closely resemble each other in many respects. Making use of the similarities, the Japanese evolved a system that is a combination of the two and that continues today to be the most popular massage method. Though their backgrounds and development processes differ, both massage and amma are today regarded as methods for relieving fatigue and maintaining general good health.

Whereas amma, based on the ideas of the tsubo and the

keiraku connecting them, tends to apply treatment first to the central parts of the body and to work outward toward the hands and feet, Western massage, which concentrates on the heart and blood vessels—in keeping with Western anatomical medical theories—begins treatment at the hands and feet and works inward toward the heart. Moreover, the effects of the two treatments differ. Traditional amma is used to relieve fatigue, stiff shoulders, heaviness in the head, sluggishness, insomnia, backaches, constipation, stiff joints, chilled hands and feet, slight swellings, etc. Western-style massage affects the nervous, muscular, and hormone systems. For that reason it is used to treat partial paralysis caused by apoplexy and in treating infantile paralysis, stiffness of the shoulders and neck, pain and numbness in the arms, weak stomach, and chronic constipation.

The reader must not think that there is any clear distinction between the realms of effectivness of the two; there is none. Primarily because the word "amma" sounds old fashioned and somewhat benighted, people lately have begun calling both methods massage. I shall use the English word throughout this book, but I shall mean by it the amma massage system based on the principle of the tsubo. I shall begin by explaining the six basic massage techniques.

Rubbing and Stroking

Placing the hands flat on the area to be massaged and pressing lightly, rub and stroke the skin. Depending on the size of the area to be massaged, it may be necessary to use only the four fingers or the thumbs or lightly to hold parts of the skin between the thumb and index finger. The most important thing to remember is to place the hands or the balls of the fingers flat on the body and to maintain unvarying pressure from beginning to end of the massage motion. Pressure is light—about three to five kilograms or only enough barely to move the needle of batroom scales with the thumb and four fingers. Because it stimulates the flow of blood and lymph, the rubbing and stroking technique relieves fatigue, improves the tone of the skin and muscles, and thus improves personal appearance. The easiest massage method to use in the home, it is effective in relieving chills in the feet and hands resulting from paralysis and slight swellings caused by obstructions in the circulatory system.

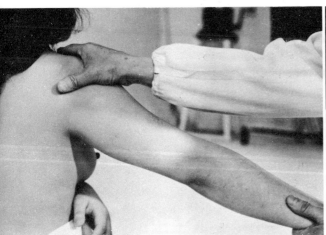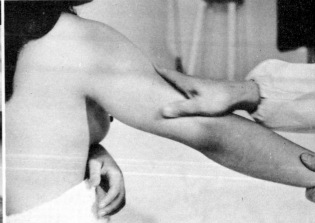

Rubbing and stroking.

Circular-motion Massage

Once again depending on the size of the area to be massaged, use either the entire palm or the tips of the fingers. If using the fingertips, grip the muscle lightly. In either case move the hands in circular motions. The circular motion must originate with the wrists, and the fingertips must not be tensed. If the motion is made with the fingertips, the patient's skin may be so irritated that it would be better never to give him a massage at all. This method relieves fatigue, improves the contracting power and flexibility of the muscles, strengthens the muscles, and relieves stiff shoulders, backaches and swollen legs resulting from fatigue. The effectiveness of this method is greatly heightend if it is preceded by thorough rubbing and stroking massage. This massage method helps develop muscle in the limbs of paralyzed children and helps remove fat from the middle aged.

Kneading Massage

Using the thumb and index finger, the middle finger alone, or all four fingers, massage the tendons crossing joints. The massage motion must be a kneading one. This breaks up pathological deposits between the elements of the joint so that they may be absorbed. In this way, the kneading massage brings relief to certain symptoms that persist after acute conditions, fever, swelling, and pain have abated following an attack of rheumatism of the joints. For instance, it helps correct enlargement and hardening that make joints difficult to bend. In addition it helps relieve semi-paralysis and stiff joints caused by apoplexy and cracking and stiff joints in people in their forties and fifties.

Pressure Massage

Once again using the palms of the hands the thumbs, or the four fingers, apply pressure—three to five kilograms—to the patient's body. The application of pressure ought to last for from three to five seconds. The secret of successful pressure massage is this. Do not press with the fingertips alone. Instead think of concentrating the entire weight of the body in the fingertips and adjust the pressure according to the body of the patient. Increase pressure gradually during one application until it reaches the maximum recommended intensity; then gradually decrease it. Direction of pressure must always be toward the center of the patient's body. Since, unlike the other five basic methods, this one supresses the actions of the nerves and muscles it is used to treat neuralgia and to cure muscular cramps. This method is basically similar to the one used in shiatsu (see pp. 27-28).

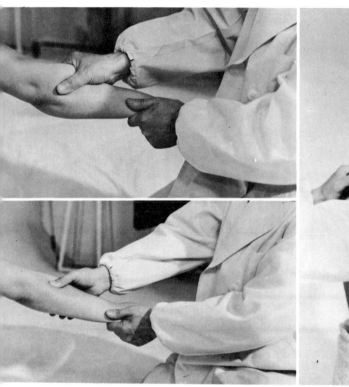
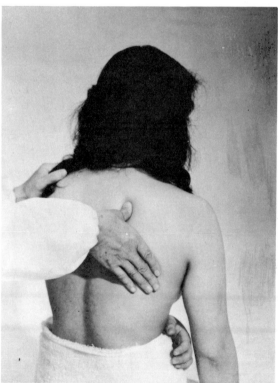

(above) Circular-motion massage.
(upper right) Kneading massage.
(right) Pressure massage.

Vibration Massage

Putting the palms or the fingers firmly on the patient's skin and pressing gently, rhythmically vibrate the hands. A skillful person can vibrate his hands from ten to forty times a second. The small rhythmical vibration improves the functioning of nerves and muscles and is therefore highly effective in relieving numbness and paralysis caused by muscular weakness or dulling of the nerves.

Tapping Massage

Using one hand at a time or both in alternation, rhythmically and lightly tap the patient's body. This may be done with the palms, the fingertips, the backs of the fingers, or with the little-finger edges of the hands. It is important to tap lightly and quickly; a skilled person can tap thirteen or fourteen times a second. Pay the greatest attention to both speed and lightness in the motion because prolonged heavy strikes affect muscles and nerves adversely. The desired effect may be achieved if you relax your fingertips, move your wrists and elbows lightly, and tap with first one hand then the other. The pressure in each tap should be about one kilogram. This method restores vitality to muscles and nerves that have become sluggish and dull. But it must be used with care, for done badly the tapping method can raise blood pressure.

After judging the symptoms of the patient's complaint, select the basic massage method that will bring maximum relief. After massage, have the patient move his joints, bend his legs and arms, raise and lower his shoulders, and bend his body forward and backward slowly.

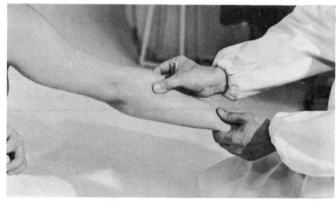

Tapping massage.
Lightly pressing the closed eyelids with the balls of the fingers.

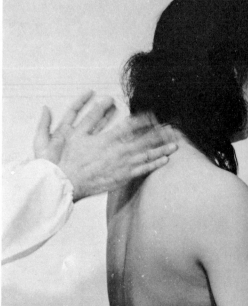

Shiatsu

The human skin is capable of three kinds of response; that of pain when it is struck by some object, thermal response to cold or heat, and response to pressure. The medicine of the Orient makes good us of stimulations to all three to correct bodily conditions. Acupuncture employs response to pain, moxa response to heat, and massage and shiatsu response to pressure. In other words, the medicine of the East, based primarily on experience, agrees with modern medicine's interpretation of the responses of the skin and has a very rational basis for therapy.

I have already discussed massage, but I should now like to give a simple description of shiatsu or finger pressure (see p. 24). Although the general tendency is to consider massage and shiatsu as the same thing, in fact, they employ somewhat different systems. Shiatsu incorporates ancient amma massage and certain judo and inducement methods that are not a part of massage. Since to delve deeply into the individual techniques used in shiatsu is beyond the scope and purpose of this book, I shall limit myself to a few remarks about proper application of pressure that are applicable to both shiatsu and other massage methods. First always judge pressure intensity by whether it stimulates a pleasurable sensation of mild pain or produces sharp pain and discomfort. Though in fact shiatsu may be divided into three general methods—spinal correction, pressure application, and exercise—it is the second branch, especially when based on the theory of the tsubo, that proves most valuable in everyday home therapy.

As in the other kinds of massage discussed earlier, so in shiatsu, the palms, the four fingers, or the thumbs are pressed against the appropriate tsubo to stimulate or depress bodily functions as the case requires. There are a variety of such application methods geared to produce differing effects in accordance with the patient's condition. In shiatsu too pressure must be controlled to suit the stiffness of the part of the body being treated.

A very important thing to remember in shiatsu pressure application is not to press with the fingertips only, but with the weight of the entire body. Pressure applied with only the fingertips merely causes pain and contributes nothing toward curing the patient. A second vital point is always to direct the pressure toward the center of the patient's body. This naturally requires that the person performing the shiatsu adopt a position that will enable him to control the pressure with his entire body and direct that pressure correctly. This depends on the part of the patient requiring treatment. For instance, if it is necessary to use shiatsu on a person's back the massager should be to the right of the patient with one knee up.

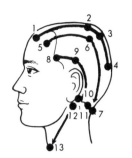

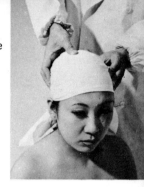

Chapter 5
Massage Treatment

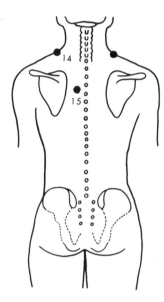

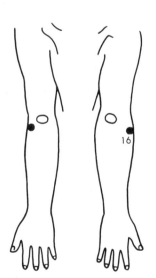

Headaches or Heaviness in the Head

Headaches may be divided into two large categories: those arising from such specific and known causes as colds, neuralgia, physiological disorders, toothache, earache, diseases inside the skull, and hemorrhage; and idiopathic headaches that are habitual and caused by uncertain factors. Of course a doctor, upon discovering the cause of a headache, can take steps to remove the cause and thus relieve the pain. But in general, most people hesitate to go to a physician for no more than an ordinary headache. The following treatment is effective for people not wishing to go to the doctor as well as for those who cannot locate the cause of their headaches.

First wrap a towel around the head and tie it securely in place at the base of the neck in the rear. The towel should be folded in half longwise. The folded edge should come well down on the forehead. This in itself frequently brings relief from heaviness in the head, but if it does not, follow these steps. The tsubo for massage are indicated by numbers on the chart.

Begin by massaging lightly at the center of the hairline (1) continue to the spots on the center top of the head (2 and 3) continue massaging at point (4) well down on the rear center line of the head. Next massage points (5) located on either side of point (1) on the hairline. Continue massaging points (6) and (7). Next beginning at point (8) continue massaging to (9) and (10) but massage in small circular motions with the palms of the hands. Now, with the thumbs of both hands, massage points (7), (11), and (10) at the base of the skull.

In case of severe headaches or aches apparently resulting from blood congestion, using the index fingers, massage points (12) and (13). The massage motions must be small and circular. When this has been done, slowly turn the face upward; the heaviness in the head will be gone. Continue the treatment, however, by pressing for from three to five seconds with either the thumbs or the four fingers of each hand on all of the points from (1) to (13).

The effect of the treatment may be heightened by massage on points (14 and 15) on the back and points (16) on the arms.

Neuralgic Pains in the Rear of the Head

Pains at the back of the head, tenseness behind the eyes, and stiff shoulders fall in this category. In the presence of such neuralgia, merely touching the hair produces a tingling pain, and the skin of the head tends to twitch or move in abnormal ways. These symptoms result from inadequate circulation of blood from the heart to the head. Excessive flow of blood produces pain because of congestion; inadequate flow, on the other hand, caused discomfort as a result of either congestion or anemia.

When the symptoms are not severe, a few simple movements of the head bring relief: bending the neck to the front, back, right, and left and slow rotation of the head. If this does not bring relief, following the keiraku shown in the chart, massage or apply finger pressure to the points in this order.

First with the palms of the hands massage the point at the top of the head (1) then the one farther down the back of the skull (2), and finally the one at the base of the skull (3). Next thoroughly massage points (4) on the sides of the head, and points (5) farther down on the sides. Next move up to points (6) roughly on the hairline at the temples then to points (7) at the mastoids behind the ears.

Use pressing movements to avoid painful pulling of the hair. Since stiff shoulders frequently accompany this kind of neuralgic pain, you can increase the effectiveness of this treatment by combining it with the massage techniques for so-called middle-age shoulders (p. 64).

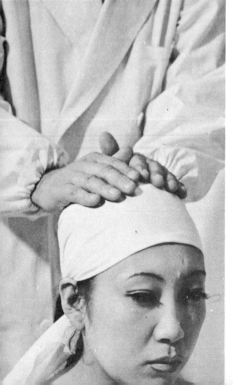

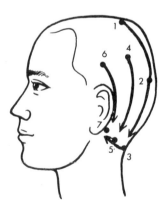

Massaging the top of the head with the palms.

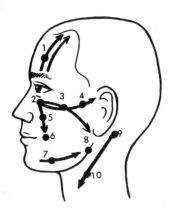

Facial Pains

This condition turns up in middle-aged people and especially women. Called trigeminal neuralgia, in its early stages it produces dull pains in the face, but as it progresses it results in sharp burning pains in the face and shoulders. In extreme cases, the afflicted person can neither speak nor eat. In addition, insomnia and extreme nervous sensitivity often characterize the condition. Although these symptoms sometimes occur with colds, diabetes, syphilis, or illness of the eyes and nose, in most cases, their causes are unknown. Since modern medical science has no treatment for them, the patient becomes emotionally insecure and sometimes neurotic.

As far as treatment is concerned, I recommend that anyone with severe symptoms of this condition consult a specialist. If the pains and manifestations are minor, however, the following massage will relieve them.

Please consult the chart. You will notice three groups of arrows—one leading from above the eyes to the forehead, one leading along the upper jaw from below the eyes to the temples and another on the lower jaw. These arrows represent the approximate keiraku of the trigeminal nerves manifesting the symptoms described above. By pressing and massaging the tsubo along these three branches, it is possible to bring relief to pain.

First, with the balls of either the thumbs or the index fingers press on the arrow leading from the tsubo at point (1). There are three keiraku below each eye; press or massage lightly in the directions shown by the three arrows on the chart. Next press on points (7) and (8) on the lower jaw. Massaging points (9) and (10) from the bases of the ears to the neck is effective too. Finally, gently stroke the whole face with the palms of the hands. In addition, comfort may be derived from heating the facial keiraku with a hot towel or the hot-air current of a hair drier.

Facial Paralysis

When on hot summer nights people sleep with electric fans trained on them, they frequently awaken with faces chilled to the point where they can neither smile nor show any other emotion.   The facial nerves become dulled by chilling or by over exertion.   In extreme cases, eyes will not close, and mouths remain so slack that food spills from them.   Under such severe conditions, the patient is suffering from a central brain ailment requiring the immediate attention of a specialist.

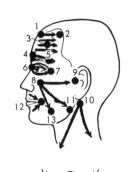

When symptoms are minor, however, it is possible to bring relief by warming the face with a hot towel and massaging with the thumbs of four fingers at the points shown on the accompanying chart.   Since the muscles that produce facial expressions are vitally important, after the massage and finger-pressure session, stand in front of a mirror and make laughing, crying, and angry faces.   Continued regularly for five or ten minutes every morning, this regimen will cure minor cases of facial paralysis.

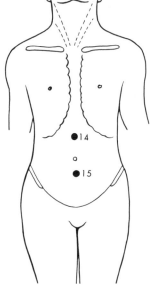

In certain instances it is also necessary to massage points (14) and (15) on the abdomen and (16) and (17) on the back. But it is most important patiently to continue both facial massage and exercises of the expressive muscles.   Do not expect a complete cure in only two or three days; it takes much more time.

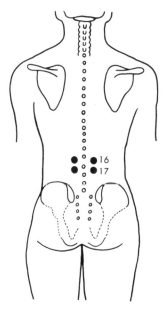

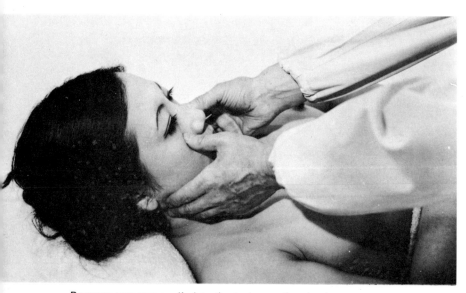

Pressure massage applied to the tsubo on the cheeks.

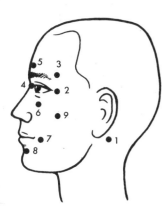

Facial Cramps

The trigeminal nerves control the ability of the face to sense heat, cold, and pain. The facial nerves govern the movement of the facial muscles. When the former are out of order, trigeminal neuralgia results. When the latter fail to function properly, the face may become paralyzed, or it may become subject to dermal cramps.

The skin of the face, unlike that of the rest of the body, is one with the muscles. Therefore, when we smile or register some other emotion with the face, both the muscles and the skin contract together at the command of the facial nerves. Facial dermal cramps result from overactivation of those nerves. Some people experience twitches or cramps around the eyes or mouth when they become angry or irritated. This condition too is the result of overactive nerves and uncontrollable muscles around the eyes and mouth.

In such cases, thoroughly massage or press spots (1) directly under the earlobe. Next, close the eyes quietly and press with the thumbs or index fingers. Follow this with applications of pressure on points (2) at the outer tips of the eyes and points (3) at the outer ends of the eyebrows. Next press points (4) at the inner ends of the eyes and points (5) at the inner ends of the eyebrows. For relief from cramps of the mouth area, in addition to points (1), massage or press points (6), (7), and (8). Pressure on points (9) relieves cramps of the forehead.

Pressure applied directly under the earlobe to relieve cramps.

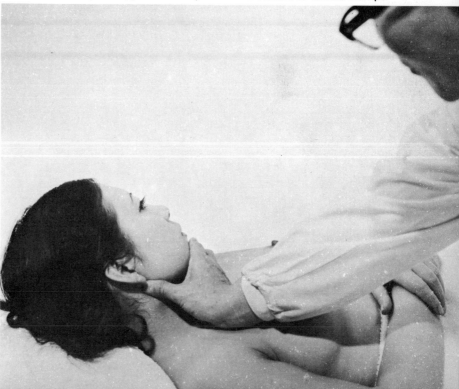

Toothache

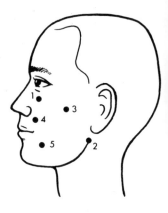

Probably most people have experienced toothache at one time or another. The causes are many, but if decay has attacked and rotted the tooth from without, the only sensible thing to do is visit the dentist to have the damage repaired. Massage can bring relief, however, to a condition caused by painful floating teeth. Either overexertion or the nerves controlling facial perception give rise to this condition.

As their name indicates the trigeminal nerves branch into three subdivisions on each side of the face. The first branch, as I have already shown, rises above the eyes; the second traverses the area under the eyes, and the third affects the lower jaw. The second branch produces pain in the teeth of the upper jaw; and the third, in those of the lower jaw. To relieve pain in teeth in the upper jaw, press or massage points (1) under the eyes. In addition, pressure with the thumbs (applied from the back to the front) on points (2) or on points (3) brings relief from pain in teeth in the upper jaw.

Pressure on points (4) just below the nostrils and points (5) below and to the sides of the mouth relieves pain in lower teeth. Sometimes pain in the lower jaw accompanies lack of sleep and headaches. In such cases thoroughly massage points (5).

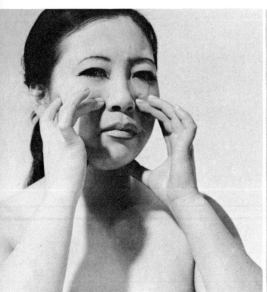
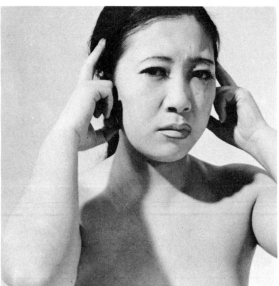

Facial massage that one may do oneself.

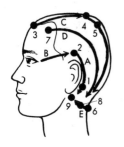

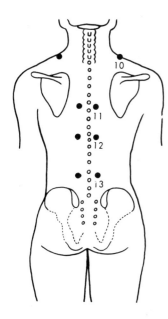

Giddiness, Ringing in the Ears, Dizziness

Lack of sleep and overwork bring on a condition in which sudden rising from a seated position causes dizziness and a metallic ringing in the ears. Generally these symptoms are caused by disorders in the ears, which assist the body in maintaining balance, or by such brain conditions as cerebral congestion or anemia, menopause, seasickness, stomach or intestinal disorders, or nervous symptoms. The condition occurs frequently in women in their forties and fifties. The following simple massage method, practiced daily, will relieve these symptoms.

Please consult the chart. There are five keiraku systems that must be thoroughly but gently massaged. First (A) centering on tsubo points (1) behind and around the ear. Next, (B) leading from the outer ends of the eyes to points (2). Now (C) leading from point (3) at the center of the hairline, through points (4) and (5) to point (6). (D) leads from points (7) at the edges of the forehead to points (8) behind the ears. Finally, (E) leads from points (6) through points (8) to points (9). Using the palms of the hand, massage each point several times gently in the order given. You may also massage each tsubo three or four times gently with the balls of the thumbs or the index fingers.

Next massage in the same way points (10) on the shoulders, (11) on the back just under the shoulder blades, (12) on the back above the liver, and (13) on the back near the kidneys. Massage points (14) and (15) on the abdomen and (16) on the sides, then points (17) on the heels, and finally the area from points (6) and (8) to the back of the neck.

Should the symptoms occur repeatedly within intervals of thirty or forty-five minutes, they suggest a condition too serious for domestic treatment; consult a specialist.

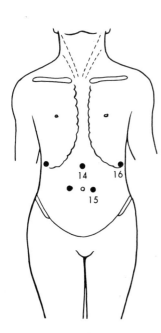

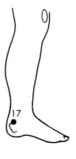

Poor Hearing

News from China that acupuncture had restored hearing to a student in a school for the deaf aroused great hopes in the parents of deaf children in Japan. But, since oriental medicine is always an individual-to-individual affair, it is never certain that a course of treatment will produce exactly the same effects in two different cases.

Deafness may be divided into two major classes, sound perception and sound transmission. Clinical experiments in our laboratory indicate that acupuncture treatment is effective only in dealing with low sounds, disorders related to which are connected with obstructions in the central nervous column. Nevertheless, Chinese medicine advocates long continuation of treatment in the hope that improvements in disordered conditions will result. Such improvement may take place if treatment of hearing difficulties is carried out long enough.

Chinese medical classics say that the kidneys control the ear. For that reason, in treating the ear we first investigate the kei system of the kidneys by checking the tsubo at points (1) and (2) on the outer side of the second lumbar vertebra, points (3) and (4) on the abdomen and sides. Further, since people with symptoms of this kind tend to have chills in the legs, it is also necessary to check points (5) and (6) inside and outside the heel and points (7) on the instep. In addition, points (8), (9), (10), and (11) on the trunk must be investigated to determine bodily condition. After this, it is possible to begin direct treatment of the ears. This is done by massaging and applying finger pressure to a number of points on the head: (12, 13, 14, 15, 16, 17, 18, 19, and 20) plus (21) and (22 and 23) at the rear hairline; these last are also used in treating headaches.

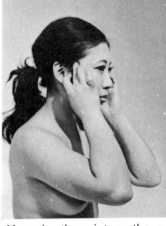

Massaging the points on the head (point 12 in this case) can be done by oneself.

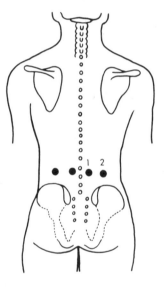

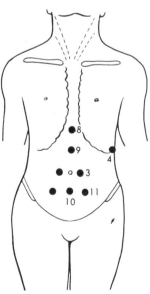

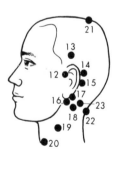

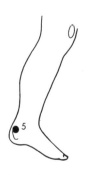

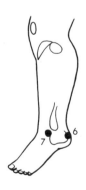

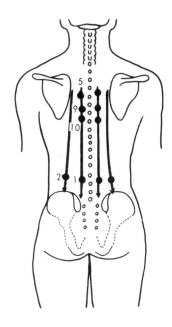

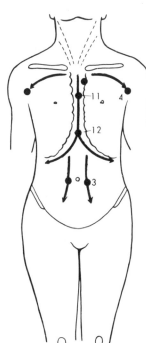

Coughs and Difficulty in Breathing

Many people complain of persistent coughs developing when autumn winds begin to blow. Though the cough may not arise during the day, when the chill of night sets in, it frequently plagues these people and brings with it large accumulations of phlegm. Still other people complain of shortness of breath following brisk walking or the climbing of a steep flight of steps. In most cases, these symptoms indicate chronic bronchitis. Once described as an occupational disease because of its prevalence among miners and workers in woolen and textiles mills, bronchitis is now becoming an environmental-pollution illness since it affects many people living in urban factory areas or near heavily trafficked highways. The symptoms can, however, arise from heart or kidney ailments or from over-drinking or over-smoking. Since severe conditions may be fatal, consult a physician. But massage and shiatsu may be used to bring relief when symptoms are light. People of poor and weak constitutions suffer from this condition.

To discover whether massage treatment is called for, press tsubo (1), (2), and (3) as shown on the chart. If pressure on these places produces pain or if the massager feels stiff areas around them proceed with the following massage. Pressure on points (4, 5, 6, 7, and 8) will relieve coughing. Massage on points (9, 10, 11, and 12) will restore normal breathing and calm palpitations. For these reasons, massage or apply finger pressure on the keiraku centered on these points. Finally be specially careful to massage points (13) and (14) on the legs where considerable stiffness may develop. All of these points may not require massage depending on the individual. To discover which ones require treatment, touch them all. Only those producing pain or manifesting stiffness will need massaging.

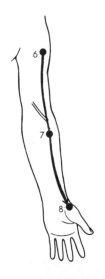

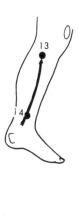

Colds

Very few people have never had a cold, attitudes toward which vary from disregard as something too trifling to require a physician to fear of the cold as the source of all kinds of other illnesses. It is a fact, however, that colds can bring on other sicknesses. And for that reason they must not be ignored. The best thing, of course, is to cure them oneself before they become serious.

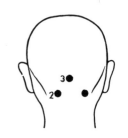

The name "cold" is generally used to describe minor respiratory ailments brought on by cold, chill, or excess moisture. From the stage in which the nasal membranes are slightly swollen, a mild fever emerges, the nose runs, and one sneezes, colds progress to more serious sore throats or to laryngitis and heavy coughing. Allowed to go unchecked, a cold may ultimately develop into bronchitis or pneumonia, at which time the services of a specialist are imperative. In this section, I am not discussing the virus-caused colds that are called influenza. But for treatment of nose or head colds, massage the following points.

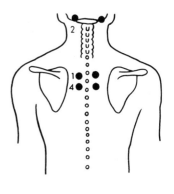

According to oriental medical theory, diseases are caused by malign influences from the exterior. The influence in the case of the cold tends to concentrate in the points shown as (1), (2), and (3) on the chart. Consequently, treatment begins with these and continues to points (4) on the back, (5) on the chest, and (6) inside the elbows. In addition to massage on the indicated tsubo, the patient must eat ample warming foods and rest well.

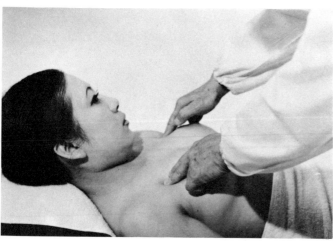

Shiatsu pressure on the chest to treat a cold.

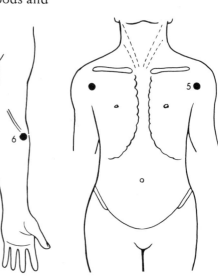

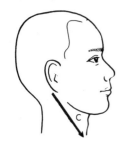

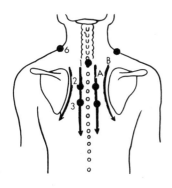

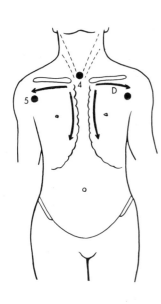

Asthma

No one who has never suffered from asthma can understand how excruciating the illness is. Breathing sometimes becomes so painful that the person cannot so much as lie down. The face drains of all normal color, and the lips turn purple. About 30 per cent of all cases of asthma occur in children of less than 10 years.

In cases of so-called infantile asthma, there are two major types: an alergy bronchitis of the same kind that afflicts adults and an asthmatic bronchitis resulting from bodily abnormalities that manifest themselves in childhood. The true causes of neither type are clear; therefore, there are no definitive treatments. Asthma is clearly a condition about whose nature many problems remain unsolved.

Just prior to or at the time of the occurrence of an attack of asthma, the patient is certain to feel pain from pressure applied to points (1, 2, 3, 4, and 5) shown in the chart. From ancient times these points have been recognized as associated with asthma. In addition to them, however, massage points (6), (7), and (8). These treatment should by repeated often. When an attack strikes, breathing can be made easier by massaging the keiraku in the directions of the arrows in the chart. The first of these starts at the base of the neck (A) and proceeds along both sides of the back to the small of the back. The second runs along the inner edge of the shoulder blade (B). The third follows the heavy muscle running from behind the ears diagonally to the side of the neck (C). In massaging these keiraku press with the thumbs and make small circular massage movements with the fingertips. Finally, pressing lightly with the balls of the four fingers, massage the collarbones (D). Soaking the hands for about ten minutes in water about 45 degrees C will relieve congestion in the chest and make breathing more comfortable.

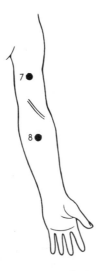

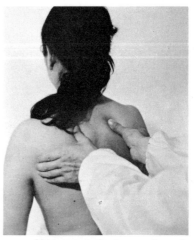

Massage on the inner edges of the shoulder blades.

Whiplash

People riding in automobiles that either crash into obstacles or are struck violently from the rear often suffer temporary sprains in the bones of the neck. This condition, now known as whiplash, results in headaches, stiff shoulders, ringing in the ears, numbness in the arms, sluggishness, heaviness, and pain in the hands and feet. The name of the sickness dervies from the whip-end motion of the neck when the automobile strikes or is struck by another object. Technically the name of the condition is vertebral sprain.

As is generally understood, a sprain occurs when a joint, that has been forced to move beyond its ordinary limits, returns to its original position. In the whiplash condition, too, one of the seven neck bones is suddenly and forcibly moved too far. When this happens the ligaments and small muscles connecting these bones are temporarily stretched. Before they return completely to normal, fever, swelling, and minor hemorrhage occur. At the same time, nerves connected with the shoulders, arms, and head are affected with the result that the patient experiences stiff shoulders, headaches, ringing in the ears, numb arms, and pain.

The neck must be immobilized for four or five days following an accident causing a whiplash condition. Then hot towels must be used to warm the ligaments and small muscles. Next, gently massage the back of the neck—arrows (A) in the chart— with the thumbs. Now, massage from the area behind the ears along the side of the neck to the collarbone (B). Massaging keiraku (C) and (D) will relieve pain in the chest. Whiplash affecting the first to fourth vertebrae gives rise to pains in the back of the neck and stiff shoulders; that affecting the fourth to seventh brings on attacks of pain in the arms and numbness and palpitations in the fingertips. Therefore see p. 64 for further information on suitable treatment.

In addition to massage, light shiatsu pressure on the tsubo shown in the chart brings relief from the whiplash symptoms.

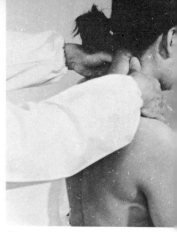

Massaging the back of the neck.

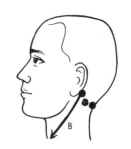

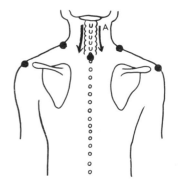

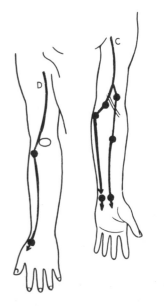

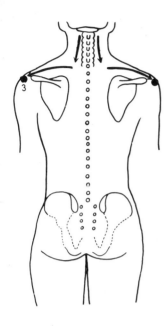

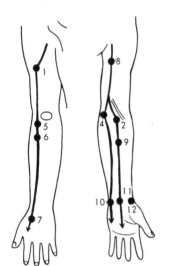

Pain in the Arms

This book deals in separate sections with the kinds of pains in the arms and back experienced by middle-aged white-collar workers who, on their days off, overindulge in house repair, golf, or other activities more strenuous than those to which they are accustomed (see pp. 63-64). In this section, however, I deal with the classic symptoms of neuralgia in the arms brought on by chill or fatigue and manifesting themselves as pain and sluggishness running from the bases of the arms, along the thumb-sides of the hand, the palms, and the little-finger side of the hands.

Neuralgia in the arms falls into three major types: radial, median, and ulnar depending on the keiraku affected. For relief from pain affecting the radius, press and massage in small circles with the thumbs from the base of the arm; these pains run from the vertebrae to the base of the neck, under the arms, along the upper and front arms to the thumb-sides of the hands. Pain affecting the median bone runs from the upper arm along the front to the center of the palm. Finally pain affecting the ulna runs from the front of the arm to the little-finger side of the hand. Heat treatment is enough to bring relief to minor symptoms. Using hot towels, thoroughly warm the neck and then, with either hot towels or the hot current from a hair drier, apply heat to the keiraku along which the pain develops.

Sometimes, however, pressure on certain spots along the keiraku will produce sharp pain. These are the tsubo that are most effective in treating this kind of neuralgia. If you massage or apply shiatsu thoroughly to points (1, 2, 3, 4, 5, 6, 7, 8, 9, 10, 11, and 12) in the chart, you will bring relief to pains of the arm.

A note of caution is in order about the nature of neuraligic pains in the arm. Sometimes muscular inflamation, poison, arthritis, or diabetes can cause similar discomfort. But though the arms will hurt, the pain will be unaccompanied by fever. In such cases, consult a physician.

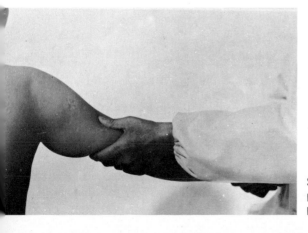

Shiatsu pressure applied to the points on the arm (point 1 in this picture) brings relief from aches.

Numbness in the Arms

Sometimes mountain climbers return from strenuous outings with heavy back packs to find that suddenly their arms are weak and their elbows are numb. When the alpinist season begins I have a number of patients—mostly young ladies—complaining of what I call the back-pack paralysis. From the base of the neck to the collarbone, around the bases of the arms, under the arms, and in the arms themselves where the straps of the pack press, these people suffer from a kind of nervous paralysis. Since in most cases the symptoms are not so severe that the nerves have altered in any way, there is little cause for worry.

Sometimes the paralysis affects the upper parts of the arms, sometimes the lower, but in either case, if the symptoms are slight, hot towels or heat treatments with a hair drier will bring quick relief. Even if massage is to be used, thoroughly heat the shoulders and arms for about twenty minutes with heat packs or hot towels. Then massage the area from the back of the neck to the outer shoulders (A). Next massage the keiraku along the inner edges of the shoulder blades (B), next the whole inner area over the shoulder blades (C) in the directions indicated by the arrows. In all instances, make kneading motions with the palms of the hands.

Now massage the front of the arm (D), the triceps (E), the biceps (F), the side of the triceps on the back of the upper arm, (G), the arm from the elbow to the thumb-side of the wrist (H), the fleshy part of the under arm (I), and the fleshy part of the arm on the opposite side (J). Massage all of these keiraku with a kneading, squeezing motion of the flat of the hand. The massage must be brisk and must follow the tsubo shown in the chart. If this does not bring relief, some aberration in the nerves themselves requires the attention of a specialist.

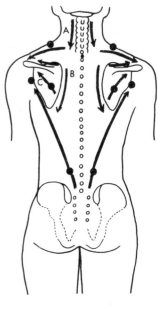

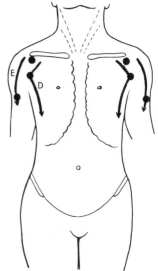

Massaging the arm from the elbow to the thumb side of the wrist.

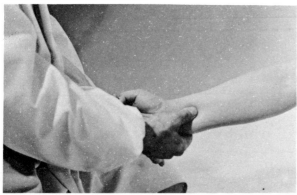

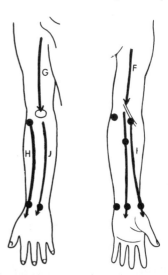

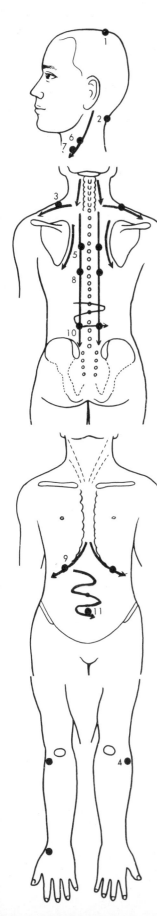

High Blood Pressure

It is difficult to judge when one's own blood pressure is high, but the condition manifests itself in such general bodily symptoms as headaches, dizziness, ringing in the ears, stiff shoulders, palpitations, insomnia, constipation, tendency to fatigue, and chills in the hands and feet. High blood pressure may be of three types: the results of kidney ailments, a symptom of arteriosclerosis, or constitutional high blood pressure. The last tends to occur in people who are psychologically unstable, frustrated, easily angered, or frequently fidgety and irritable. Since it plagues businessmen in executive positions, high blood pressure is sometimes called the managerial illness. Persons in the forties or fifties must avoid excesses in all activities for this is the period of life in which blood pressure changes.

Of course, if there were a single tsubo on the body that, when pressed or massaged, would immediately lower blood pressure, the problem would be simple. Unfortunately, however, there is no such tsubo. Consequently, the therapy for high blood pressure consists in treating each of its symptoms one by one. Because headaches, stiff shoulders, and heart palpitations always accompany the situation, begin massaging points (1) and (2) on the head and (3) on the shoulders. Next treat points (4) on the inner sides of the elbows, points (5) on the back, and points (6) and (7) on the neck keiraku. For patients unable to sleep at night, massage points (8) on the back and (9) just under the rib cage. For those who are easily tired, massage points (10) on the back and point (9) between the navel and the pubic region. For patients with chilled hands and feet, to the treatment described above, add shiatsu pressure to points (12) and (13) on the feet and ankles.

Massage all of the keiraku along which the tsubo listed are located; follow the arrows. Have the patient lie facedown and lightly tap the plantar arches (14) with the fists about one hundred times each. An electrical vibrator too will prove effective in stimulating the plantar arches. This treatment will bring about an amazing lowering of the blood pressure and a refreshing of the general bodily condition.

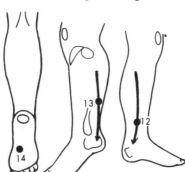

Tap or use an electric vibrator on the plantar arches.

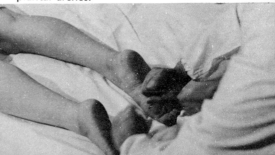

Low Blood Pressure

It is possible to estimate a person's optimum blood pressure by adding 90 to his age. A maximum pressure of less than 100 is considered low. Although many things may cause this condition, in general low blood pressure may be divided into three main types: symptomatic low blood pressure, rising low blood pressure, and constitutional low blood pressure. Prolonged confinement in bed as a result of poor nutrition, heart disease, or tuberculosis causes the symptomatic variety; when the basic condition is relieved, blood pressure returns to normal.

In the condition with the somewhat peculiar name "rising low blood pressure" it is not the pressure, but the person, who rises. This condition develops often in thin young women. As long as they remain lying down, their blood pressure is normal, but it drops when they get out of bed. At such times, they become victims to attacks of dizziness and giddiness. But the most common kind of low blood pressure is constitutional, which is, in fact, the result of uncertain causes. Tall thin people with poor appetites, constipation, generally poor physiology and the appearance of anemia are prone to this condition. Such people tire easily and rarely stay with a piece of work for a long time. Although their symptoms are similar, anemia and constitutional low blood pressure are the results of different causes; for that reason, always verify the nature of the condition of the patient by consulting a physician before launching on a course of home treatment. If the trouble is ascertained as contitutional low blood pressure, begin therapy by having the patient eat plenty of foods rich in proteins and fats.

In order to return the body to normal working condition, massage or apply shiatsu pressure to the following tsubo. Begin with treatment of the tsubo on the head: points (1) and (2). To correct dizziness, ringing in the ears, and giddiness see p. 35; for weak stomach and gastritis see p. 46. Treat for fatigue and chills in the hands by massaging points (3), (4), (5), and (6). Massage on points (7), (9), and (10) is effective in relieving chills in the feet. Incidentally, in our clinic, ultra-short wave, supersonic wates, infrared, and ultraviolet treatments have proved effective in curing low blood pressure.

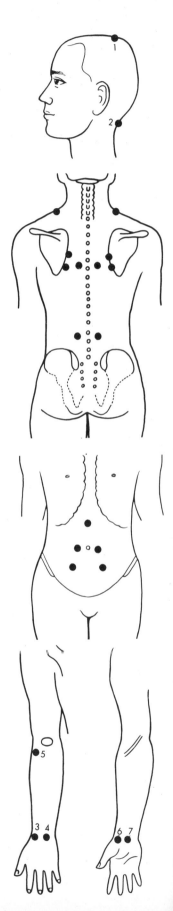

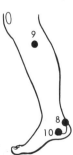

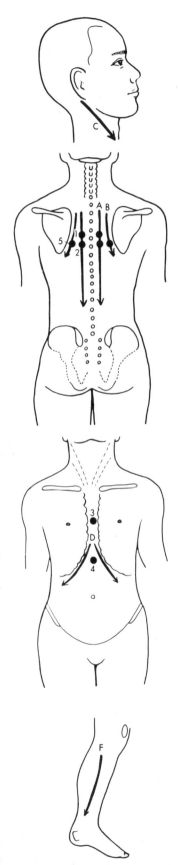

Heart Palpitations

Many people, especially nervous women between their thirties and forties, complain of sudden unexplained heart palpitations in the middle of the night. Once the attack begins, they are unable to go back to sleep. They soon become uneasy and first experience pain around the heart and then alternating chilling and sweating. If thorough professional examination reveals nothing wrong with the heart itself, the patient is probably suffering from a condition known as heart neurosis or nervous heart and brought on by prolonged periods of irritation, anger, or insecurity. Psychological treatment, tranquilizers, and sleeping medicines have been used against the condition, but as a result of their side effects, medicines are now being abandoned in favor of psychological and physical—especially oriental medical—treatments that both bring relief from the palpitations and effect a general return of harmony to the body functions.

Important tsubo for massage in treating this condition are points (1) and (2) on either side of the fourth and fifth thoracic vertebrae, point (3) located on the chest between the breasts, and point (4) at the diaphragm. In addition, massage on points (5) at the inner edges of the shoulder blades is effective in this connection. The arrows from (A) to (F) indicate the directions of massage. Following them, massage the vicinity of each tsubo thoroughly.

Since this condition is difficult to cure completely, it is important to combine the attention of a specialist with home treatment. Avoid stimulants like coffee, alcoholic drinks, and tobacco.

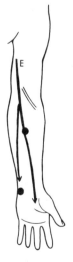

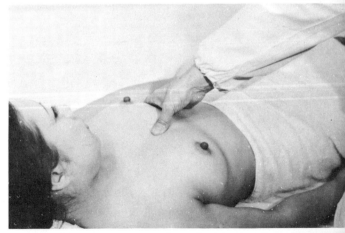

Shiatsu pressure on the tsubo between the breasts.

Chronic Gastritis

Poor appetite, periodic sharp pains or heaviness in the abdomen, sour belching, heartburn, and nausea are produced by inflammation of the stomach lining and chronic gastritis. When they become severe they indicate a condition demanding thorough investigation, stomach photographs, and x-rays by a specialist. Before they reach such a stage, however, they may be treated in the following way.

From ancient times, oriental medicine has advocated the efficacy of moxa used on six spots related to the stomach: points (1), (2) and (3) on the right and left sides of the back. Massage too on these points is effective in treating stomach ailments. In fact, the stiffness and tension that develop there when stomach trouble occurs substantiate the idea of their usefulness in treatment of such illness. I have already commented on the connection between internal disorders and their surface manifestations and on modern medical opinions concerning this points (see p. 19). In the case of gastritis, the heavy muscles on which points (2) and (3) lie are especially important as are points (5) just inside the shoulder blades. The keiraku that must be massaged in treating this ailment are (A), which runs from the shoulder blades (5) down the back to the hip area (3), (B), running from the diaphragm outward to each side and along the lower edge of the rib cage (6), (C) leading from the diaphragm to the navel (7), and (D) passing through points (8) on each side of the navel. Using the palms of the hand and working in the numerical order shown on the chart, massage these keiraku in the directions of the arrows. When treating the points on the back, make small circular motions with the balls of the thumbs.

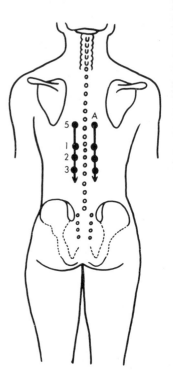

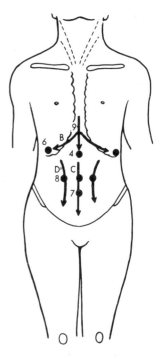

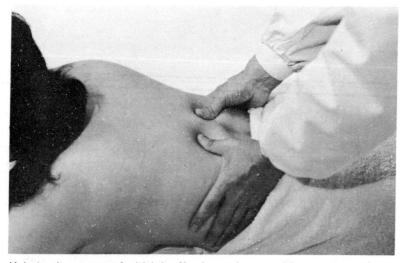

Keiraku A, massage of which is effective against gastritis, begins under the shoulder blades.

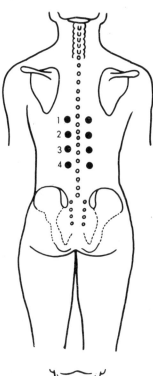

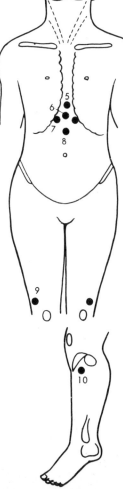

Stomach Cramps

Spasmodic attacks of pain in the abdomen, called stomach cramps and today referred to as nervous symptoms, range in severity from mild to violent and in duration from one or three minutes to one or two hours. The pain affects the area from the diaphragm to the sides. Causes include the physical and the nervous. Cramps may arise from the consumption of tainted food, from indigestion, gallstones, stomach or duodenal ulcers or from overactivity of the nerves traversing the stomach. In addition, constriction of the stomach walls causes cramps. Organically caused cramps require the attention of a physician, but milder symptoms may be treated at home with massage and shiatsu pressure.

The tsubo at points (1, 2, 3, and 4) located next to the seventh, ninth, tenth and eleventh thoracic vertebrae are important in treating this condition. Point (5) at the lowest tip of the sternum, point (6) on the diaphragm, points (7) next to the ribs, and point (8) are the central zones for massage with the thumbs or the four fingers, or for shiatsu pressure.

When an attack strikes, warm the stomach while massaging the tsubo on the back and abdomen listed above. After the cramps have eased, stretch out the patient's legs and apply shiatsu pressure to points (9) above the knee caps and to points (10) on the sides of the shins. When this treatment is completed, the patient will feel so much better that his earlier suffering will seem no more than an illusion. Since these cramps attack people who are nervous, general calm in daily life is a good way to prevent their occurrence.

Using four fingers to apply pressure to points in the diaphragm area.

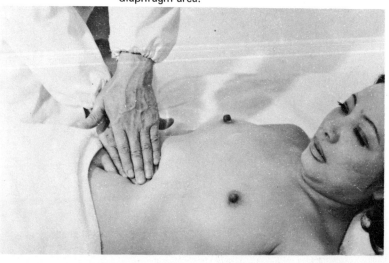

Pains in the Chest and Sides

After strenuous work or exercise or after a cold, people often suffer from excruciating pains running from the left side of the back along the side of the body or along the sides at about the height of the nipples. Breathing or talking with a loud voice makes the pain seem to reverberate throughout the entire body. A slight bending of the body toward the unaffected side brings on stronger, virtually unendurable pain.

Because broken ribs, caries of the bone, and cancer of the chest produce similar symptoms, consult a physician at once when this kind of pain occurs. If thorough checks show that there is nothing seriously wrong, if there is no fever, and if x-rays reveal nothing, you may be assured that the pain is caused by the nerves between the ribs. Since the eleventh and twelfth ribs are not attached to the sternum, strong external impact can twist them thus delivering shock to the nerve roots and causing neuralgic pains between the ribs. In such cases, have the patient lie on one side, with the side in pain upward. After applying hot towels to the area in pain and rubbing it lightly with the hands, massage the keiraku shown in the chart.

Beginning at points (1, 2, 3, 4, 5, and 6) on the back, massage in the directions of the arrows. Next, using the balls of the four fingers, press (about three kilograms of pressure) points (7, 8, 9, 10, and 11) on the chest and upper abdomen. Now have the patient sit up and while breathing deeply insert his hands under his armpits, arms crossed on chest, and raise his arms and shoulders quietly five or six times. This treatment should gently stretch the nerves into normal position and relieve the pain. In cases of very light symptoms, hot towels or the warm current from a hair drier may be sufficient to bring relief.

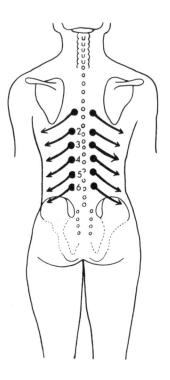

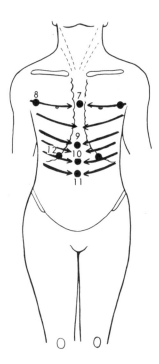

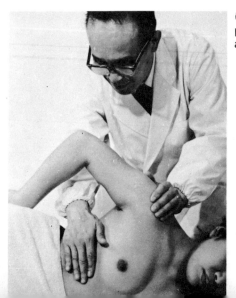

Using the balls of the fingers, press the chest and upper abdomen.

Backaches

The causes of so-called backaches are numerous. Pain in the back may result from disorders in the bones, joints, or ligaments, neuralgia, chill, colds, or female troubles. Sometimes, however, urinary-tract and stomach and intestinal diseases manifest symptoms of pain in the back. Because of the multitude of possible causes, even trained specialists find making accurate first diagnoses difficult. Obviously the untrained amateur cannot determine the causes of backache with any accuracy. For that reason, in this and the following sections, I present ways of curing the symptoms without reference to the causes. According to oriental medical theory, if the symptom is cured, the cause of the trouble will naturally have been eliminated. This section deals with persistent backaches and the following with sudden sharp pains in the back.

The usual backache, which is severe in the morning when the patient first arises and gets better as he moves about, will show no reactions in x-ray or blood-precipitation tests. The condition is difficilt to analyze and understand. Although it responds to hot baths expecially in salt hot-srings or sulfur-springs water, a total cure is not to be expected. Relief from pain may be achieved, however, by first heating the areas around the tsubo shown in the chart with hot towels for about twenty minutes. Next, placing the left hand on top of the right and using the palm of the right hand, massage and press keiraku (A). Continue to massage keiraku (B) and (C) making small circular motions with the palm of the hand. Now apply shiatsu pressure with the thumbs to keiraku (D) working in the directions indicated by the arrow.

Finally massage the buttocks—keiraku (E)—making large circular motions with the palms of the right and left hands. To strengthen the stomach muscles, massage and apply shiatsu pressure to the tsubo shown on the abdomen.

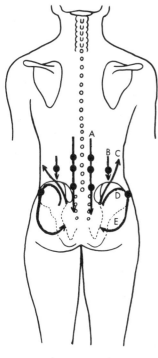

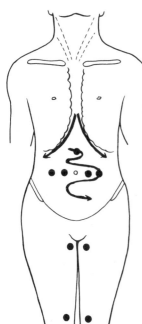

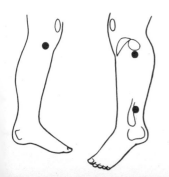

Circular action used in massaging the back and buttocks.

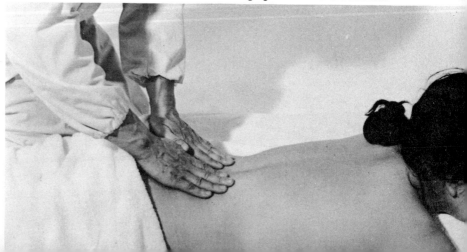

Sharp Back Pains

Unlike the more or less steady pains described in the preceding section, the sharp back pains treated here usually occur when a person bends or attempts to lift something. If severe, they make it impossible to stand straight.

An acute affliction, these pains most often result from dislocations or malformations in spinal discs. The conditions are commonest in people of middle age or more. Back muscle sprains too can be the cause. This is the case with many young men who fail to get proper exercise because they spend too much time riding in automobiles. When they do engage in some energetic activity, they sprain their backs and bring on these sharp pains.

Before massaging the tsubo, touch the part of the body that is in pain to determine whether there is fever or swelling. If there is no fever, apply hot towels and have the patient lie still for about twenty minutes. Use cold towels if there is fever. Next have the patient lie on his back, as you apply shiatsu thumb pressure instantaneously and simultaneously on points (2) on both feet. Continue to apply similar pressure on points (3) and then on points (4) on the back of the calves.

Next, have the patient lie on his stomach. Centering the massage motions on the points (5, 6, 7, 8, 9, and 10) and, following the arrows, massage both sides of the small of the back and downward toward the buttocks. Take special care to massage the places where the patient feels pleasurable sensations.

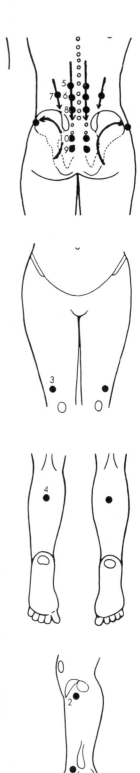

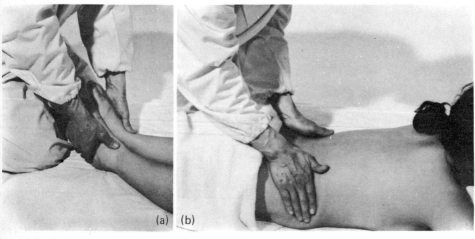

(a) (b)

(a) Simultaneous and instantaneous pressure on tsubo 1.
(b) Pressure or massage applied on the tsubo from the small of the back toward the buttocks.

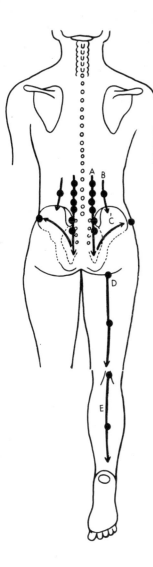

Back and Leg Pains (Deformed Lumbar Vertebrae)

Pains in the back and legs are frequently caused by deformations in the cartilaginous discs among the lumbar vertebrae or by deformations resulting from age in the vertebrae themselves. A similar condition caused by deformation of the knee joint is said to be as common in middle-aged women as balding is in middle-aged men. Since the causes in vertebral conditions are aging, returning the patient's condition to normal is difficult, but massage can bring relief from pain.

The first step is to apply hot towels to the back in the area from the first to the fifth lumbar vertebrae and the first to the third sacral vertebrae. Next massage thoroughly the areas located at keiraku (A), (B), and (C) on the chart. Next heat—with hot towels or a hair drier—the backs of the thighs (D), the backs of the calves (E), the insides of the knees (F), and the sides of the knees (G). Massage these same zones in the directions of the arrows.

When the pain in the knees is severe, remember to heat them with towels and, after thorough massage, have the patient sit so that his legs dangle without touching the floor and execute some light leg-limbering exercises.

Patients, who had been suffering from this condition for many years, are cured completely after a course of from two to four months massage three times weekly. But be careful to avoid chilling and over-exertion, which can bring the condition on again.

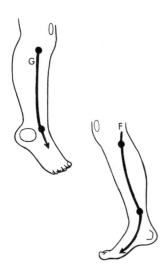

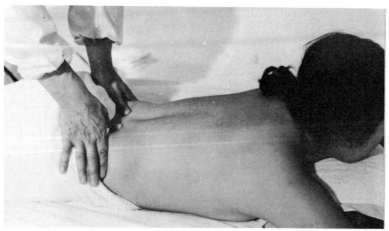

Through massage on keiraku (A), (B), and (C).

Back and Leg Pains (Sciatica)

Sciatica is characterized by these symptoms: pain is not apparent when the body is at rest, but coughing, hiccoughing, or bending produce pains that run from the waist through the buttocks, the backs of the thighs, and the calves. Sometimes the pain extends as far as the heels; sometimes it begins in the outer sides of the ankles and runs to the insteps. If one raises one's legs with the knees straight, severe pain will arise in the lower legs. The sciatic nerve, the thickest nerve in the body, runs from the back, through the buttocks, thighs, and legs. When the kind of pain described occurs, however, always have a physician investigate thoroughly since disorders in the spine and spinal chord, diabetes, pelvic diseases, and pressure caused by cancer can produce the same symptoms.

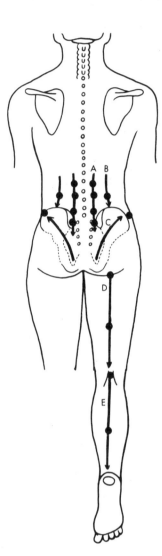

If the cause is only age, however, relief may be obtained by applying hot towel packs for about twenty minutes and massaging thoroughly. Areas to be massaged are keiraku (A) and (B) running along the heavy muscles on either side of the backbone, keiraku (C) in the buttocks, keiraku (D) running down the center of the back of the thighs, keiraku (E) running from the back of the calves to the plantar arches, keiraku (F) running from the outer lower leg to the ankle, and keiraku (G) running along the front of the lower leg. In massaging these areas, work in the directions of the arrows and use the palms of the hand. In addition, shiatsu thumb pressure on the indicated tsubo is effective. When applying shiatsu, use from three to five kilograms of pressure for from three to five seconds on each tsubo.

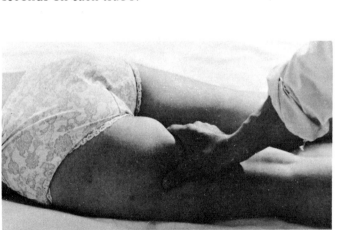

Massaging the keiraku running down the centers of the backs of the thighs.

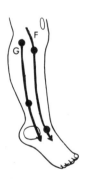

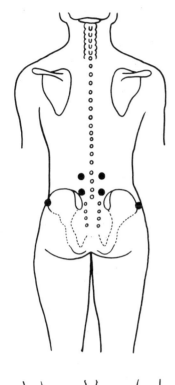

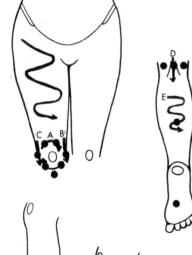

Pain in the Knee

As I mentioned earlier, many middle-aged women, especially the overweight, complain of pain in the knee when they rise from chairs or go up and down steps. This is caused by deformation of the knee joint accompanying advancing age. Early symptoms of the condition are chill, swelling, or accumulation of liquid on the knee and pain and cracking sounds made when the joint is moved. When the knee hurts, the body tends to shift the load this joint generally bears to the back, thighs, and calves with resulting pain and heaviness in these now over-burdened muscles and bones. In this section, however, I shall concentrate on treatment for pain and swelling in the knee only.

To improve blood circulation and thus relieve discomfort quickly, apply hot towels to the knee for from twenty to thirty minutes. Then for about five or six minutes every morning, noon, and evening, massage the knees, thighs, and calves as shown and in the order indicated in the chart. First, using the thumb and fingers of both or of only one hand, thoroughly massage keiraku (A) in the vicinity of the kneecap. Continue massaging keiraku (B), (C), and (D) in the same way. Then in kneading motions with the flats of the hands, massage the calves (E) and the large muscle of the thighs (F). Persistent and careful massage done in this way for two or three weeks will bring relief.

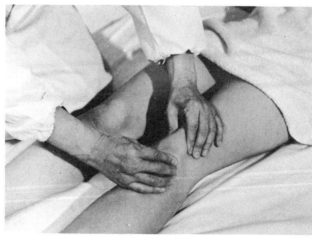

Massage the vicinity of the kneecap with the thumbs and fingers.

Cramps in the Calves

Sharp, tearing pains in the calves often attack while people are sleeping. The only thing to do then, unless one knows how to apply quick relief massage, is to grip the aching muscle and hope for the agony to pass. Instead of an actual sickness, these pains are physiological phenomena occurring as a result of two conditions. They tend to develop in sick people whose recovery is not progressing as well as it should or in healthy people who are very tired after an unusually energetic bout of mountain climbing, swimming, or some other strenuous exercise. It is very wise to learn the places to massage and the tsubo to use in applying shiatsu pressure, because no one can tell when these painful cramps will strike.

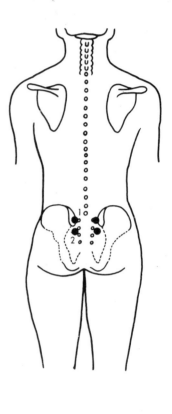

Signals delivered by the brain while one sleeps set the nerves in the calves into overaction, which in turn tenses the calf muscle causing the pain known as cramps. Shiatsu is more effective than massage in calming the nerves: the human tendency to grip the muscle and press it when it is in a cramp condition indicates the efficacy of this treatment. Apply plenty of pressure with the fingers to points (1) and (2) at the small of the back and then to (6) and (7). Next press (3), (4), and (5) on the back of the knee, the back of the calf, and the place where the calf muscle joins the Achilles tendon. These three are most important and deserve special attention. Using the thumbs and fingers, first press lightly then increase the pressure. Each application must last from three to five seconds. This shiatsu therapy works with amazing speed. And its effect can be improved by bending the big toes back as far as possible several times.

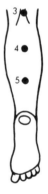

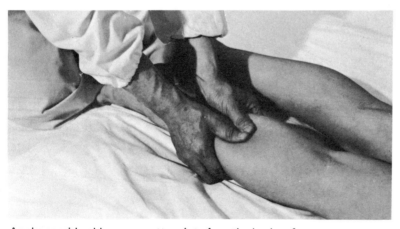

Apply considerable pressure to points 4 on the backs of the calves.

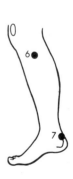

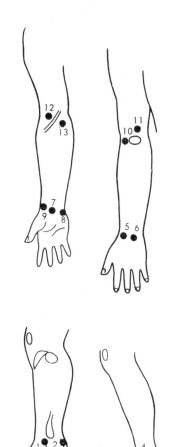

Rheumatism of the Joints

Sometimes pain in the joints comes from overexertion and fatigue, but persistent aching joints early in the morning, stiffness, and a tendency to swell may well be signs of rheumatism. This sickness usually begins with the small joints and progresses to the larger ones. Its symptoms are especially noticeable at times of seasonal change or in wet weather. The joints gradually become painful and stiffen; in extreme cases, they harden entirely and lose the ability to move at all. The disease occurs especially in women of more than twenty years of age. When it becomes chronic it is extremely difficult to cure. Children who manifest symptoms of rheumatism are generally victims of rheumatic fever, which frequently attacks the heart.

Though many people suffer from rheumatism of the joints, no complete explanation of its causes has yet been forthcoming, and oriental therapy is still the best method of bringing relief. The basic principle of this therapy stated briefly is improvement of the blood circulation of the entire body. The very name of the disease derives from a Greek word meaning a flux or flow, and indeed it does flow throughout the body manifesting its symptoms in first one joint then another. Once again, warmth, including hot packs and if possible paraffin baths, is recommended. Daily massage on the areas around the tsubo in the charts (1, 2, 3, 4, 5, 6, 7, 8, 9, 10, 11, 12, and 13) will bring relief.

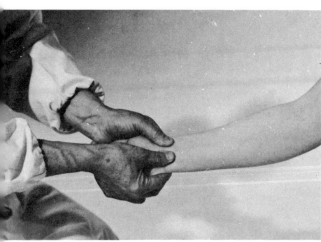
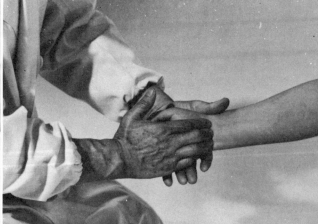

When massaging the wrists, refer to these photographs and duplicate the method shown.

Allergy

Localized or generalized itching, rash, and swelling that characterize allergic attacks may be of the sudden kind that passes in a matter of days or weeks at the most, or they may be chronic and persist for months or even years.

Many people are allergic to foods, flowers, or certain kinds of climate. Their allergic reactions may take the forms described in the preceding paragraph, or they may manifest themselves internally in tired eyes, nose colds, stomach or intestinal disorders, cramps in internal membranes, or even bronchial asthma.

People with allergies frequently have rashes or dry, scaly areas on the back in a triangular area running from the base of the neck to the outer edges of the shoulders. Pressure applied with the thumb to the seventh cervical vertebra—located at the level of the tops of the shoulders—produces sudden sharp pain. Repeated massage at point (1) will greatly reduce the appearance of allergic symptoms. Massage on points (2) on either side of the third thoracic vertebra, points (3) on either side of the ninth thoracic vertebra, points (4) on either side of the second lumbar vertebra, and points (5) on either side of the fourth lumbar vertebra, plus point (6) in the middle of the chest, point (7) on the diaphragm, point (8) below the navel, and points (9) on each wrist will heighten the effect of the massage.

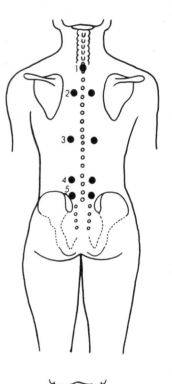

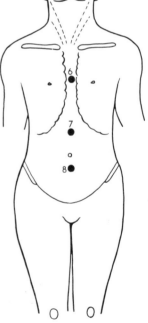

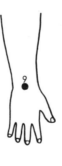

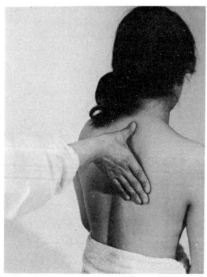

Massaging points on either side of the third thoracic vertebra.

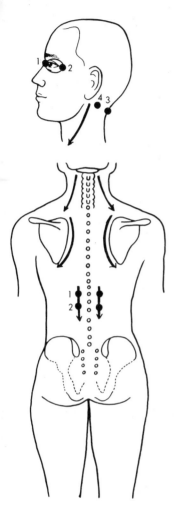

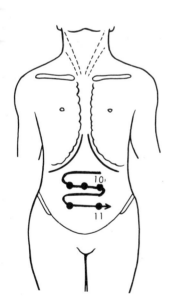

Diabetes

Classic symptoms of this disease—sometimes called the beginning of all illnesses—are unexplainable weariness, dry mouth, and a tendency to lose weight no matter how well one eats. At the appearance of these conditions, consult a physician immediately for thorough examinations. People of middle age who lead irregular lives involving numerous parties and too much drinking tend to develop diabetes. The condition is characterized by an accumulation in the blood of sugar, which fails to function efficiently as a source of energy, and by inadequate insulin secretions from the pancreas. In order to relieve the condition by stimulating efficient use of blood sugar, it is necessary to supplement the body's insulin supply. Shiatsu pressure and massage are obviously powerless to effect this part of the cure, but they can bring relief to certain diabetic symptoms.

Dry mouth and tendency to lose weight result from an inadequately active pancreas. Consequently, massage on points (1) on the back and on points (2) below them on either side of the twelfth thoracic vertebra stimulates this organ and improves digestion and breathing.

When the other diabetic symptoms are accompanied by forgetfulness and headaches, massage points (3) and (4). Massage on points (5, 6, 7, 8, and 9) is effective in relieving sluggishness in the arms and legs. Treat points (10) and (11) for constipation. Massage must center on these tsubo and must be performed in the directions indicated by the arrows.

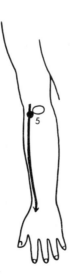

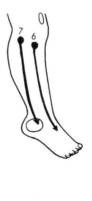

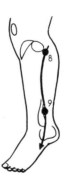

Bedwetting

Few parents today consider scolding and spanking suitable treatment for a bedwetting child. The following information will be useful in discovering the cause and bringing about a cure for this condition. Generally the lower bodies of children who wet the bed tend to be chilled. In addition, infant sufferers from bronchial asthma—and their number is increasing in modern cities—often wet the bed. Finally, there are some children who do this as a result of irregular living patterns and bad habits. These latter two causes are beyond the immediate curative possibilities of massage, but chilled lower bodies can be successfully treated by massaging the following tsubo.

Point (1) located between the navel and the pubic bone and point (2) just at the edge of the pubic bone are effective points for treating both infantile and adult bedwetters. In addition, points (3) directly to the sides of the second lumbar vertebra and points (4) to the outer sides of these, points (5) on either side of the second sacral vertebra, and points (6), (7), and (8) for the sake of chilled legs require treatment. Points (9) beside the nails on the outer side of the big toes improve the functioning of the liver and thus relieve chills. Either massage or shiatsu pressure on these tsubo will bring results.

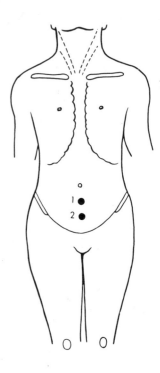

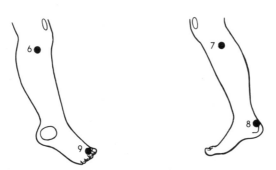

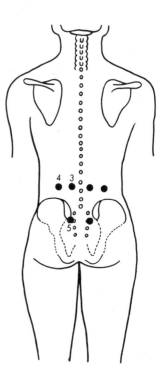

Night Weeping

In the modern urban environment of cramped spaces, pollution, noise, and continual dinning of the radio and television, children are sometimes made so nervous that the cry late at night. If this condition is not cured, it can develop into hysteria. The most important tsubo for massage in dealing with night weeping is (1) on the spinal column. In fact, this point has long been considered of major importance in dealing with all infantile sickness. But since it is difficult to find exact intervertebral locations on the bodies of children, follow this procedure. Starting just below the hairline on the back of the neck, lightly press or rub the skin along the spine toward the shoulders. When you strike a certain point the child will suddenly twitch. Press gently in this vicinity and when you find a spot at which the child makes a definite response, you will have located tsubo (1). Continue treatment by lightly rubbing or pressing points (2), (3), (4), and (5). Obviously, one must never use great pressure in treating small children. But with continued gentle massage of the kind outlined above, the child will gradually calm down and stop crying.

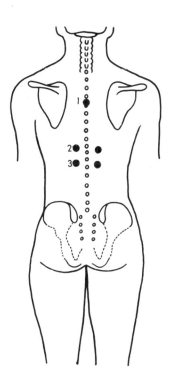
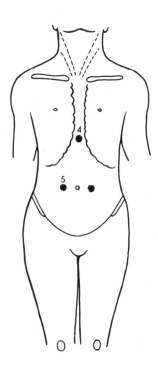

Irritability

Calm can be restored to angry and irritable children by massaging points (1) for the location of which see the preceding section, and (2) on the spinal column, points (3) on either side of the ninth thoracic vertebra, point (4) on the sternum, point (5) between the diaphragm and the navel, and point (6) below the navel. In the Orient, acupuncture with special instruments modified and reduced in size for the treatment of children has long been used to sooth bad tempers, but massage on the points listed here works just as well.

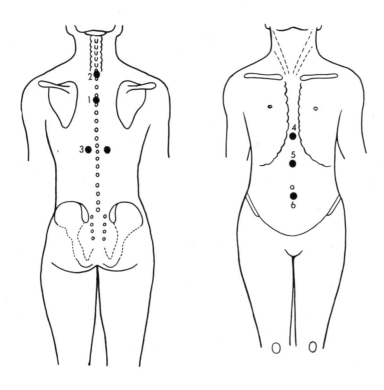

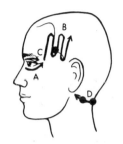

Chapter 6
Massage for General Well Being

Tired Eyes

In the whirlwind of moving vehicles, flashing neon, too many advertisements, and other distractions almost everyone today suffers from stinging eyes, glare, pain or heaviness behind the eyes, stiffness in the back of the head and neck, and general sluggishness. A few minutes of massage as outlined below after long sessions of reading or other close work will refresh both the eyes and the whole body.

Lying on your back, lightly close your eyes. Using the thumbs or the four fingers, massage or press the areas on the edges of the eyes along keiraku (A) shown in the chart and in the directions of the arrows. Do not press directly on the eyeballs. Instead direct the pressure to the bones around the eyes. Begin with light pressure and gradually increase it. Next, moving the four fingers of each hand, lightly massage in a circular fashion keiraku (B) between the outer edges of the eyes and the areas in front of the ears. Now with the balls of the four fingers of each hand, lightly press on the closed eyelids (C). Apply pressure for from ten to fifteen seconds and gently remove the fingers. Finally, massage the bone at the base of the skull with the balls of both thumbs in the directions shown (D).

In addition to this treatment, relief from stiff shoulders can be had by massaging keiraku (E) and (F) on the back and shoulders.

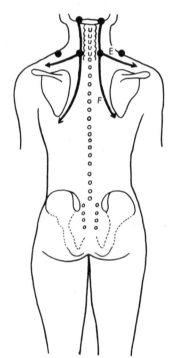

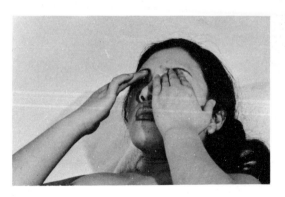

Insomnia

Of the currently increasing number of people who awaken too early in the morning, cannot sleep soundly at night, or find that they sleep in positions that later cause stiffness or other pain, many are suffering from a nervous condition, others are victims of high blood pressure or stomach or intestinal disorders. Before attempting the therapy described here, carefully read the sections on these conditions and make an effort to put the entire body in good physical condition. Remember that a person suffering from insomnia frequently compounds his affliction be being afraid that he will not be able to sleep. Calm and composure are essential to sound rest. Consequently, the patient must not aggravate his nervous state; even if he cannot sleep for one or two nights it will have no serious effect on his health.

People who cannot sleep are almost always stiff in the part of the back shown at tsubo (1, 2, 3, and 4) in the chart. Massage there can do much to bring relief. Furthermore, their abdominal region (tsubo 5, 6, 7, 8, 9, 10, 11, and 12) is usually so tense that slight pressure brings discomfort and firm pressing sharp pain. This area too requires treatment, but massage must be light and performed with the thumbs in the directions shown by the arrows. It must be executed in the numerical order indicated by the tsubo numbers.

If sluggishness in the legs or feet is the cause of the insomnia, massage as shown on p. 65. A beer bottle rolled lightly over the muscles of the leg and the bottoms of the feet, especially at tsubo (13), brings relief. Chill in the feet is often the source of this trouble. For that reason, the patient must take care to keep his feet well covered at night.

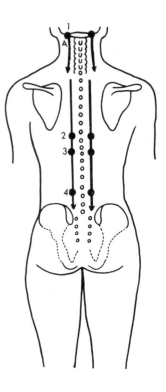

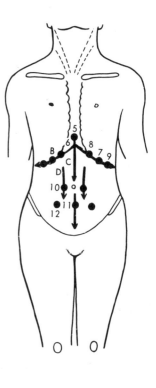

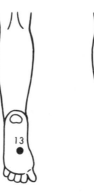

Pain and Numbness in Neck, Shoulders, and Arms

People in early middle age sometimes awaken with stiff wrists and numb fingertips. This is the result of symptoms affecting the neck shoulders and arms. The cause is disorder in the seven cervical vertebrae that support the weight of the head or in the cartilaginous discs among them. This disorder exerts pressure on the blood vessels and nerves leading from the head to the neck, shoulders, and arms and thus causes heaviness or stiffness in those parts of the body.

When these symptoms develop, lightly press or tap the neck in the area of the cervical vertebrae (see chart). Tsubo (1) will be the place where tapping produces pain. Begin treatment by immobilizing and warming the neck for about twenty minutes. Next, using the four fingers of both hands lightly press and rub keiraku (2) and (3) in the directions of the arrows beginning at the base of the skull and working up to the area behind the ears and downward toward the base of the neck. Continue by massaging thoroughly keiraku (4), (5), and (6) which cover the entire area between keiraku (2) and (6). This will prove amazingly effective, but results are even better if you gently press each of the points shown on the chart with the thumbs. In massaging one's own neck and shoulders, one tends to move only the fingers. For greater effect, attempt to move the arms from the shoulder blades.

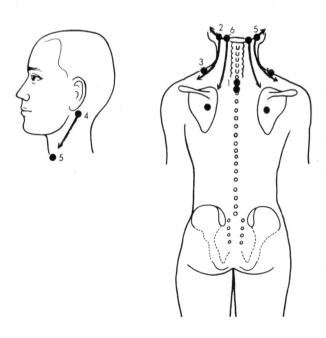

Middle-age Shoulders

Actually an inflamation of the bone around the shoulder joint, this discomfort—called fifties shoulders in Japanese—is characterized by chilling, a feeling of heaviness, and pain. People in their forties and fifties are often afflicted with it. If allowed to reach an advanced stage, it can make movements of the hands and arms very painful and can make it difficult to lift the arms or bring them behind the body.

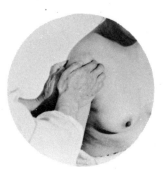

Massaging keiraku (C).

A similar condition may be caused in younger people by wounds from the outside of the body, but in the elderly it is usually the result of disorders in the muscles, tendons, and ligaments around the shoulder caused by ageing in the joint. In accordance with the oriental medical principle of heating chilled areas and cooling feverish ones, middle-age shoulder requires the application of hot towels since it tends to produce chilling. Once the joint is completely warmed, using the flat of the hand, lightly but thoroughly massage keiraku (A), (B), (C), and (D). You will find that this treatment gives surprising results.

An additional highly effective treatment involves the use of a fairly heavy clothes iron. Holding it in the hand of the arm that is in pain, bend forward, and swing the iron back and forward in wide arcs.

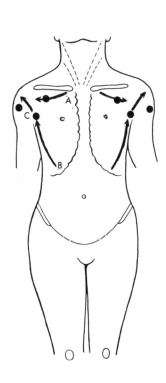

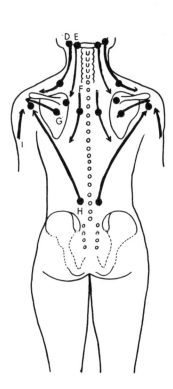

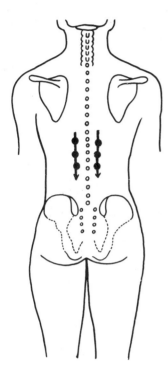

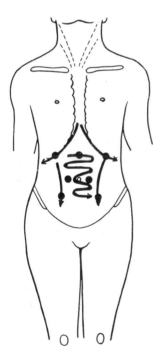

Poor Appetite

Healthy people generally experience increases in appetite with the approach of autumn. Throughout the summer, when a large percentage of the blood flows near the surface of the skin, one is rarely very hungry, but in the fall, when the blood tends to flow in greater quantities around the inner organs, appetite ought to return. People whose stomachs and intestines have not recovered from the weariness caused by summer heats, however, often fail to experience this.

But loss of appetite may be caused by other conditions as well: nervous tension brought on by over-work, lack of sleep, worry, or frustration, and such physical ailments as gastritis, stomach or duodenal ulcers, stomach cancer, constipation, parasitemia, or anemia. For that reason, it deserves the attention of a specialist. If thorough examination reveals no physical cause and thereby suggests that the loss of appetite is caused by nerves, over-work, or constipation, apply the following oriental treatment. Shiatsu pressure on the tsubo shown in the chart and thorough massage on the keiraku indicated by the arrows will stimulate appetite by calming the nerves, improving digestion and respiration, and eliminating excess gas from the body. In using shiatsu pressure, work lightly but prolong the duration of each application.

Since the pleasures and values to be derived from good food are of the greatest importance to health and happiness, perform this massage daily. In addition, eat plenty of nourishing food and make every attempt to ensure that the appearance of the foods is appetizing.

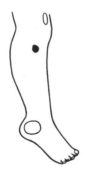

Sluggishness in Legs and Back

One has only to realize that the legs support the body's weight, make walking and running possible, and preserve bodily balance to realize their importance. Modern science has shown that the lower part of the back too is of the greatest significance largely because the adrenal glands are attached there. When these glands fail to function, the effect is felt all over the body. Conversely when the body is in generally poor condition, the adrenal glands become sluggish. As the legs and back show no signs of weariness, the body can go on working for some time, but when they begin to grow tired, the whole body will soon be desiring to rest.

Prolong periods of standing or sitting can make the legs and feet swell by impairing blood circulation. In such cases, more exercise is recommended, but massage and shiatsu pressure too can be useful.

In the center of the plantar arch is a tsubo (1) that oriental medicine has long valued as a barometer of health for if this spot is stiff the legs will require treatment for chill or for weariness or stiffness.

Begin the treatment by applying hot towels or hot packs to the back especially from the small of the back to the buttocks. The application should last for from twenty to thirty minutes. Next apply shiatsu pressure to points (2), (3), and (4) and massage keiraku (A). Follow this by massaging keiraku (B)—from tsubo (5) to tsubo (6)—with the palms of the hands. Continue by massaging keiraku (C), (D), and (E) in the directions of the arrows.

Rolling a beer bottle back and forth over the plantar arch while seated in a chair brings relief from tired feet.

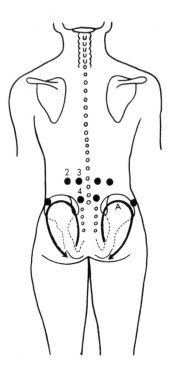

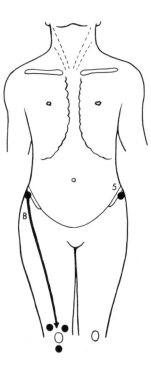

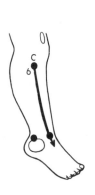

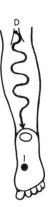

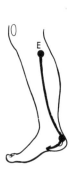

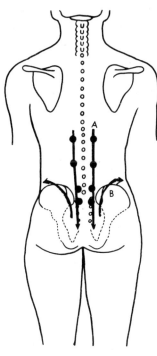

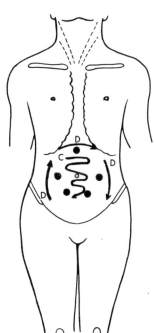

Constipation

Although physical causes such as illness of the stomach, intestines, or sexual organs, pregnancy, bodily characteristics, or irregular living cause constipation, nervous strain and the diet too play an important part. It is difficult to set a limit on what is normal and what abnormal in bowel movements, which differ with individuals.

In general disorders in the autonomic nervous system produce either sluggishness or hypertension in the intestines and thus cause constipation. Home remedies involving massage and hot packs are effective only in dealing with constipation resulting from sluggishness. Consult a physician for treatment of intestinal hypertension.

First have the patient lie facedown and using the palms of the hands and making small circular motions with the thumbs, massage keiraku (A) along the spine and (B) to the outsider sides. Next have the patient lie faceup. Placing the left hand on top of the right, massage keiraku (C)—from the navel to the top of the pubic region—(D)—to the right and left sides of (A).

Instead of massaging, it is also possible to apply what amounts to shiatsu pressure only with the small end of a beer bottle on the tsubo shown in the chart. The effect will be greater if the bottle is full.

If this regimen is repeated daily, regular habits maintained, and the body suitably exercised, constipation should clear up soon.

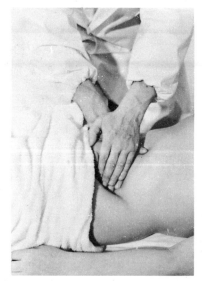

Massaging the abdomen with both hands.

Menstrual Irregularity

In a multitude of cases physiological disorders arise from such psychological conditions as worry, sorrow, changes of residence, or shifts in the weather. Women are especially susceptible. Such conditions influence the interbrain which governs emotional reactions, ovulation and the secretion of hormones from the anterior lobe of the pituitary gland. If these secretions are abnormal, ovulation fails to take place as it ought; that is, it occurs irregularly at either longer or shorter intervals than the normal two weeks. Sometimes women suffering from such disorder menstruate more often than usual and sometimes they go for as much as six months without menstruation.

The three things that must be done to restore this function to normal are these: ample nourishing food, regular habits and rest, and correction of the hormone secretion disorder. Massage and shiatsu pressure on tsubo (1) and (2) will help effect the last, as will thorough massage on tsubo (3, 4, 5, 6, 7, and 8). Heaviness and dizziness of the head frequently accompany menstrual disorder. In such cases, massage and pressure on points (9, 10, 11, 12, and 13) are effective. Since chilled feet too are a symptom of this condition, be especially careful to keep the feet warm and if necessary sleep with stockings on.

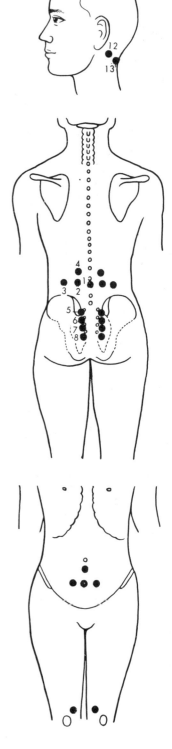

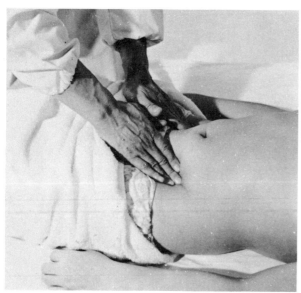

Massage on the unnumbered points below the navel too helps relive this kind of irregularity.

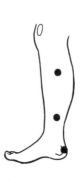

Impotence

Two major causes explain the current claim that impotence is on the increase. First, modern society is more publicly conscious of sexual activity than in the past; consequently, people pay more attention to this kind of trend. Second, the complicated stresses of contemporary civilization exert great influences on all aspects of human psychology and physiology, and the sex organs and sex related emotions are among the most susceptible to such influences.

Of course, physical illnesses and disabilities as well bring on this condition; for example failure of the penis to function as a result of automobile accident damaging the brain or spine; chemical poisoning resulting from habitual use of alcohol; sleeping medicines, or stimulants; diabetes, or obesity. Conditions of this kind naturally require the attention of specialists, but the overwhelming number of cases of impotence are those arising from uncertain psychological causes. These can be cured by means of oriental therapy, especially massage and shiatsu pressure.

Before beginning any treatment, however, one must improve one's environment. But since this is often difficult to do, it is sometimes necessary to begin by adjusting one's own mental state. Massage daily for three or five times on each of the following tsubo will be extremely helpful in doing this and consequently in curing impotence: tsubo (1, 2, 3, 4, 5, 6, and 7) on the back and buttocks; tsubo (8, 9, 10, 11, and 12) on the abdomen and inner thighs; and tsubo (13) and (14) on the legs and ankles.

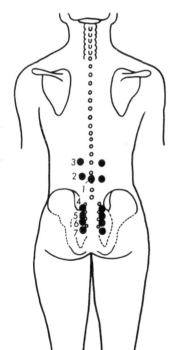

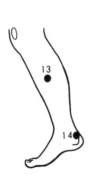

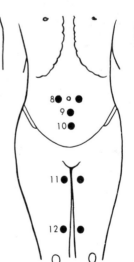

Improving Sexual Powers

Although the treatment described here will increase performance ability in the sex act, it is primarily intended as a treatment to develop general strength and to promote mental and spiritual health. As the reader will by now have learned, oriental medicine concentrates on the preservation and efficient use of both the energy the human being is born with and of the energy he receives from the world of nature after birth. If this energy flows through the body in abundance, sexual powers are great, but they fail as this energy decreases. For this reason, to increase sexual power oriental therapy advocates massage on the tsubo that govern the flow of innate and acquired energies.

These are tsubo (1, 2, 3, and 4) on the back; tsubo (5, 6, 7, 8, 9,) on the abdomen, tsubo (10) on the ankles; tsubo (11) on the inner thighs; tsubo (12 and 13) on the inner sides of the knees; tsubo (14) on the calves; tsubo (15) on the upper sides of the wrists; and finally tsubo (16) on the plantar arches. Before beginning treatment, press firmly on tsubo (7) beside the navel. If this area is stiff or if pressure produces sharp pain, it is a sure sign of failing sexual powers. Next massage in the order given above.

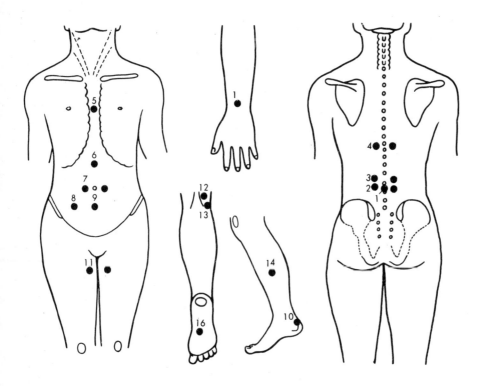

Chapter 7
Cosmetic Massage

Beautifying the Skin

No matter how smart a woman's clothes or how fashionable her hairstyle, if her skin is scaly, dry, and lusterless all of her efforts at beautification will have been wasted. A balanced and correct secretion of natural oils and sweat keeps skin smooth, soft, and lustrous. The nerves controlling these secretions are the same ones that run from the chest and around the abdominal organs. Keeping them in top condition ensures good skin.

According to Chinese medical theory, tsubo (1) on either side of the second lumbar vertebra govern the innate physique and energy of the body. Interestingly enough, modern science locates the suprarenal glands, the most important of the secreting glands, at this spot and thus endorses what therapy by experience long ago asserted. Food is the source of postnatal energy; the tsubo (2) on either side of the first lumbar vertebra control the absorption of nutrients from that food. In addition, tsubo (3, 4, 5, and 6) control the general condition of internal organs and the distribution of nourishment. Consequently, people with poor skin—a definite sign that the total bodily condition is under par—will notice marked improvement if they first heat the areas around these tsubo and then massage or apply shiatsu pressure to them regularly.

In addition, accumulation of gas and constipation are serious causes of poor skin. To the treatment described above, add those for these conditions (see p. 67).

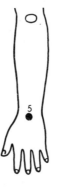

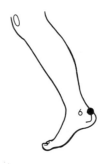

71

Removing Facial Wrinkles

Even women who take extremely good care of their skin develop wrinkles after they pass the age of about thirty. This is unavoidable since, as I mentioned in the section on facial cramps, the skin and muscles the face are a single unit. Small wrinkles develop most readily in areas where the muscle layer is thin and the movements of the face small and frequent. For instance, the ends of the eyes, the forehead, and the neck directly under the chin are cases in point.

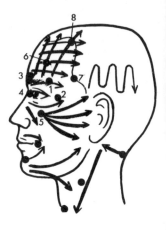

Unlike the face, the covering of the top of the head consists of separate layers of skin and muscle. Since it is the connecting point between these two different zones, the forehead is most likely to wrinkle. As the face may be considered to extend to the collarbone, careful treatment of the skin of the neck to is necessary to prevent wrinkling.

Once wrinkles have formed, however, use the following methods to remove them. For those around the eyes, apply shiatsu pressure to or massage tsubo (1, 2, 3, and 4); these are the ones used in treating facial cramps too. While applying pressure to these points, massage the eyelids and the area below the eyes and the area leading from the point under the eye (5) in the directions of the arrow; that is, across the cheeks and towards the ears. To remove wrinkles from the forehead, massage the areas shown by the arrows centering on point (6). Using the fingertips, rub in the directions shown by the arrows toward the hairline and toward the temples. In addition, massage from the hairline toward the ears in an area centered on tsubo (8).

Continue by massaging in the directions shown by the arrows from points on the upper and lower lips. For wrinkles in the neck, again work in the directions of the arrows; raise the chin and spread the hands wide while massaging. Center the massage on the tsubo shown. When you perform the massage yourself, rub the right side of the neck with the left hand and vice versa.

At the conclusion of massage, stand in front of a mirror and exercise all the facial muscles.

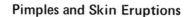

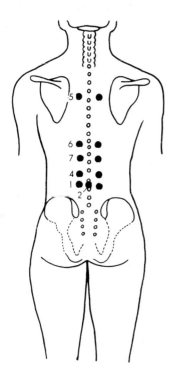

Pimples and Skin Eruptions

Although considered a symbol of adolescence, pimples are caused by a variety of complicated factors. They may result from too much or too little hormone secretion or vitamins. They be caused by digestive or atonomous nervous disorders. People with oily skin tend to develop them easily. Sometimes they are the result of bacterial infection. In young people they occur as red risings on the face, arms, and back. These bumps fester, and pus emerges. In very serious instances they leave black marks. But this kind of pimple generally is not a cause of extreme concern, since it generally passes after puberty is over. Instead of concentrating on ways to remove the pimples themselves, oriental medicine strives to prepare the body to make the transition from childhood to adulthood smoothly.

The most important tsubo for massage to achieve this transition are (1) on either side of the second lumbar vertebra and (2) on the vertebra itself. Slowly but firmly press this latter; sometimes merely touching this point restores the body's energy to a normal state of activity. In this connection, one must not forget tsubo (3) and (4) since they improve digestion and respiration. Massage and apply pressure to tsubo (5, 6, and 7) to revitalize the skin and muscles. Massage tsubo (8, 9, and 10) as well since they are deeply connected with the liver and the spleen, for centuries believed to control the condition of the skin and muscles.

Take steps to prevent constipation—a great cause of pimples—by following the procedures described on p. 67. Finally, massage or shiatsu pressure on tsubo (11) on the wrist is effective in treating carbuncles and boils.

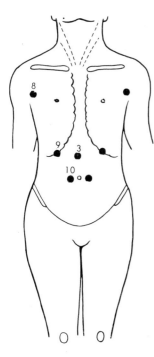

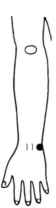

Freckles and Skin Stains

Called liver spots, these stains on the face, especially around the eyes and mouth, turn up often in young ladies just past puberty, and they a source of great concern for women of middle years. Their causes are numerous: the ultraviolet light of the sun, mental or physical over-exertion, pregnancy, women's sicknesses, malfunctioning of the suprarenal glands, liver trouble, etc. For stains with known causes, consult a physician, and in all cases avoid direct strong sunlight and lead a regular life including plenty of sleep. Freckles, on the other hand, may be hereditary. If they are very conspicuous consult a physician, but once again for fair people with light skin who tend to freckle easily, a good word of advice is to avoid strong sunlight.

Unfortunately, oriental medicine has no cure for freckles, but for the sake of total bodily health which may be effective in clearing them up, massage tsubo (1, 2, 3, 4, 5, and 6). Consulting the chart, massage and apply shiatsu pressure in the areas around these tsubo. In addition tsubo (7) on the wrists and (8) on the heel are effective in this connection. It is a good idea to massage areas that freckle easily or to stimulate them lightly with the point of a toothpick. In some case this stimulus to the skin is enough to remove freckles and stains. Modern medicine uses bleaching creams and adrenal hormones.

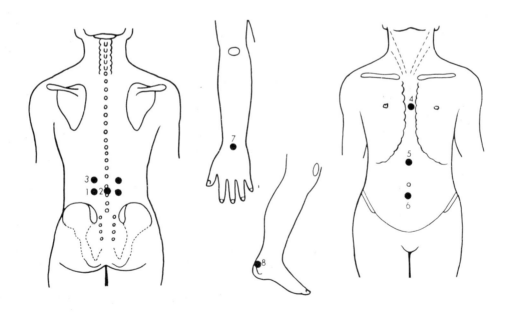

Beautifying the Eyes

Instead of applying eyeshadow and other cosmetics to attempt to create a bright-eyed appearance it would be wiser to place more emphasis on restoring the natural gleam and luster to one's eyes. Obviously regular living habits and a minimum of night work and other taxing exertion for the eyes are ideal, but this is not always possible. In this section I will explain how to use massage to refresh tired eyes and return to them their natural sparkle.

First lightly close the eyes then press them gently with the palms of the hands for about ten seconds. Remove the hands suddenly. Press again. Repeat this procedure four or five times. Beginning at tsubo (1), gently press the eyes with the thumb. Continue pressing all the way across the lids. Repeat this procedure on the lower lid but use a slightly thrusting action of the index, middle, and fourth fingers. Repeat this several times. Next, using the index, middle, and fourth fingers, massage tsubo (2) in small circular motions. Apply shiatsu pressure and massage to tsubo (3) and (4) on the neck.

Women will find that their appearance greatly improves if they perform this regimen daily before putting on their makeup.

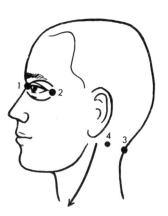

Beautifying the Voice

In order to avoid misunderstanding, I must say at the outset that I do not pretend that massage is able to change the nature and quality of the voice a person is born with. What can be done, however, is to restore to its original condition a voice that has grown weak as a result of general physical debility or one that has altered its pitch because of sickness.

Ancient Chinese medical theory involving the Fu and Zo internal organs (see p. 5) holds that alterations in these organs produces changes in the voice. Obviously, from any medical standpoint, the respiratory organs are important to the voice. In addition, the kidneys must be in good condition, if the voice is to have optimum quality.

In order to keep these organs functioning smoothly, massage tsubo (1) located on the right and left of the third thoracic vertebra and tsubo (2) located on each side of the second lumbar vertebra. Massage on these points will restore vigor to a weakened voice. To improve the beauty of tone of the voice, massage tsubo (3) on the neck, (4) on the base of the thumb (5) on the inner sides of the arms, (6) on the shoulders, and (7) on either side of the navel.

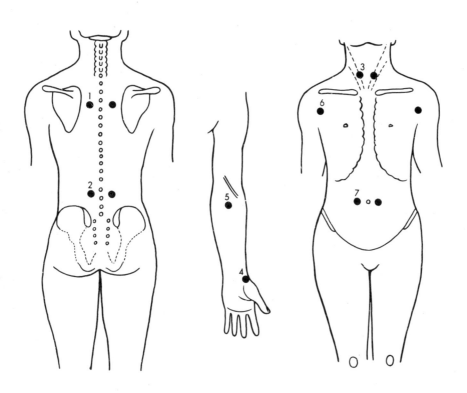

Losing Excess Weight

It is difficult to say how much weight is too much, but there are a number of charts showing average and ideal weights for ages and sizes. Consult these, and if you weigh more than you should, follow the procedures outlined here.

In the human body excess fat tends to collect on lines from the sides of the chin to each nipple, on the belly below the navel, on the inner thighs, behind the kneecap, and at the ankles. One is overweight if too much fat is present in these places. Using either the palms or all the fingers massage the areas around the tsubo shown in the chart. Pay special attention to the soft areas between the muscles. It is not a good idea to become thin to the point of emaciation; simply remove excess. Of course regular habits, balanced diet, and plenty of sound sleep are important parts of any weight-losing program.

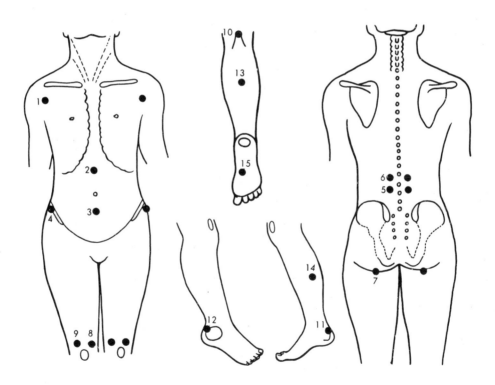

Slenderizing the Waist

Much of human appearance is a result of heredity and can therefore be altered little. But the waistline is generally large or small depending on eating and exercise habits. For that reason, many people in their middle years—both men and women—devote a great deal of attention to trimming off as many excess inches as possible. Obviously, effort can prevent the waistline from expanding, and even after it has spread, more effort can return it to normal.

Waists get big for one or both of two reasons: abdominal muscles weaken and sag or fat accumulates on the belly. Tightening the muscles of the abdomen both reduces waist dimensions and gives fat less room to accumulate. Massage daily tsubo (1, 2, 3, and 4) on the abdomen and (5) and (6) on the back. In addition perform exercises for the abdominal muscles, keeping these tsubo in mind all the time. Some good exercises are bends, leg-lifts, and situps. The effect of this massage will increase if it is performed after a good sweat in a sauna.

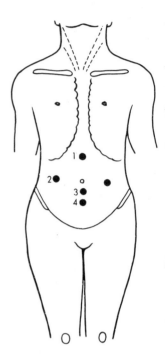

Situps help keep the waist slim.

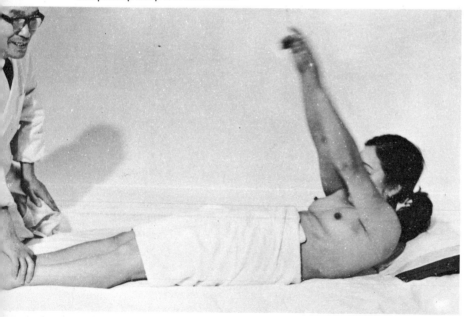

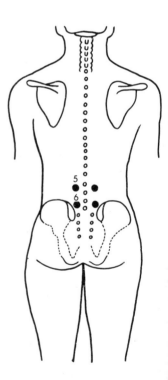